D1292864

It All Started with Hippocrates

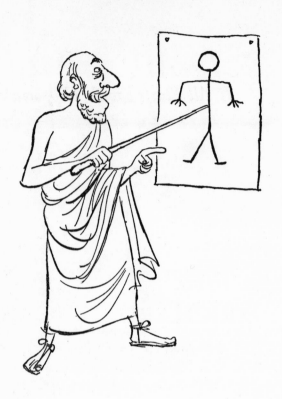

It All Started with Hippocrates

A MERCIFULLY BRIEF HISTORY OF MEDICINE

RICHARD ARMOUR

with Illustrations by Campbell Grant

McGRAW-HILL BOOK COMPANY

New York   Toronto   London   Sydney

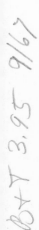

Acknowledgments

The germ (and I use the word advisedly) of
this book can be detected in "A Mercifully
Brief History of Medicine," which first appeared in JAMA (*Journal of the American
Medical Association*). For suggestion of the
original article and encouragement and
guidance during its expansion into a book,
occasionally prescribing a stimulant and
about as often prescribing a sedative, I am
grateful to my friend and medical mentor
Lester S. King, M.D., Senior Editor of
JAMA.

CONTENTS

It All Started with Hippocrates

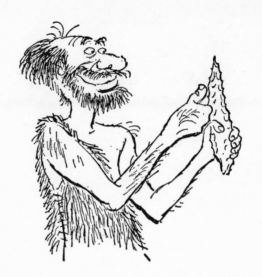

Chapter One

MEDICINE IN
PREHISTORIC TIMES

Medicine began with the dawn of history. In fact it began shortly before dawn, at about 3:00 A.M., when the first Stone Age doctor was routed from his bed to attend a patient who thought he was dying. Transportation being none too good (this being before the invention of the wheel), by the time the doctor arrived the patient was well.

During the Stone Age the most common complaints were gallstones, kidney stones, and stumbling over stones. Some complaints could be heard for blocks.[1] There being no telephones, the doctor had to be summoned by going to his cave and knocking. Since knocking on the mouth of the cave made no sound

[1] There was nothing wrong with people's lungs, since no one smoked cigarettes.

and knocking on the stones around the mouth of the cave was hard on the knuckles, it was often necessary to resort to some other way of getting the doctor's attention. The usual way was to throw a stone into the opening. If it lit near the doctor, he would hear it and know someone needed help. If it hit the doctor, he would need help himself.[1]

The doctor's little black bag was at first a little brown bag, since it was made of tree bark. A doctor with a friendly bedside manner often made a joke of this as he entered the sickroom. "My bark is worse than my bite," he would say, thereupon laughing so uproariously that it was hard to believe he had used the same witticism as an ice-breaker on six previous calls that day.

Despite the difference between the color of the bag used in those early days and the one used today, a precedent was set that still survives. Before leaving to make his calls, the doctor carefully filled his bag with every possible medical item, omitting only such things as he later discovered he needed desperately.

Some doctors had their office in their home—in other words, in the same cave or in a small cave attached to the main cave but with its own outside entrance. They could write off this part of their home as a business expense, even though it could also be used as a guest bedroom.[2]

[1] In those days, a doctor who was stoned wasn't drunk. He had, however, received a summons.

[2] The word "office," it should be noted, derives from the opening of a cave. A Stone Age patient would say, using the word in its original form, "I am going to the doctor's orifice."

Most doctors, however, had their office in a cave downtown or in a medico-dental cliff, honeycombed with caves. Since there were no old magazines,[1] the doctor's waiting room was an even drearier place than it is now. Patients had nothing with which to divert themselves, and often sat there for hours, whittling a soft stone with a hard stone. For the most part, though, they passed the time much as they do today, looking furtively at the other patients and wondering what was the matter with them.

Patients about to be examined were asked to disrobe. This was easy, because it simply meant slipping their bearskin or tiger skin suit[2] over one shoulder and letting it drop. If the nurse took their weight,

[1] Indeed, there were not even any new magazines, left there by mistake.

[2] The sharkskin suit came later.

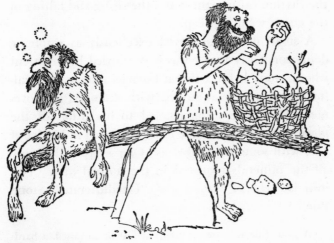

British system

she used the British system, announcing to the doctor that the patient weighed so many stones.

One striking difference between the practice of medicine in the Stone Age and today was that in those early days big strong men never fainted at the sight of a hypodermic needle. Had they seen one, however, they probably would have. As it was, they fainted only when the doctor showed them his bill—a primitive but effective type of anesthesia.

Having no stethoscope, the Stone Age doctor was forced to place his ear directly against the patient's chest. This was not easy, if the patient was a male, because of the thick growth of hair which not only muffled sounds but in some instances pierced the doctor's eardrum. If the patient was a female, however, there was no trouble, though a doctor occasionally listened and listened and finally, lulled by the rhythmical heartbeat and the rising and falling of the chest, went to sleep.

A small flat stone served excellently as a tongue depressor. Only rarely was it swallowed by a patient who mistook it for a throat lozenge. Accidental swallowing of small flat stones, with dramatic improvement of various ailments, led to invention of the placebo. Stones also came to be dispensed in bottles of 100, with some such label as "One a day will supply all the minerals required in the normal diet." The initials "U.S.P." stood for "Unadulterated Stone Pile." [1]

---

[1] A stone pile was not, as might at first be surmised, a hardened hemorrhoid.

Not until near the end of the Stone Age were chocolate-covered stones available for children and others who had trouble getting plain ones down.[1]

The Stone Age hospital was in a large cave which, however, was never quite large enough. Wings were always being excavated, as soon as they could be financed, to provide single caves and double caves and ward caves for people who needed around-the-sundial nursing care.

Surgery was in its infancy, largely because of the difficulty of making an incision with a sharpened stone and performing a suture with a stone needle. When a surgeon decided not to operate, everyone breathed a sigh of relief, especially the surgeon and, if he was still breathing, the patient.

One of the most popular operations was trepanning, as is indicated by the number of skeletons found with holes in their heads by archeologists.[2] Why so many holes are found in the occipital region is a matter of controversy among medical historians. Some think it was to let the evil spirits out. Others think it was to let the evil spirits in, the skulls being used for drinking cups. Still others think the holes were made because of brain disorders, especially on the part of surgeons who had an obsession about seeing what was inside and couldn't wait for the invention of X-rays.[3]

[1] Once a stone went down, though, it stayed down.

[2] This originally read, "skeletons found by archeologists with holes in their heads," and it still reads more smoothly that way.

[3] They learned their technique from plugging watermelons.

A prehistoric skull has been found in Peru which shows five distinct perforations. The surgeon must have been looking for something, and refused to give up. Or possibly someone told the patient he had a good head for music, and he went to the doctor and asked to be made into a flute.

In the Neolithic Age there was a great advance in surgical instruments. In addition to sharpened pieces of flint there were now thorns and the teeth of fish and animals. When a surgeon laid out his instruments, preparatory to an operation, the patient usually took a quick look and fainted dead away, making anesthesia unnecessary. However, the anesthetist stood by with a large club in his hand, ready to take care of the patient if he showed signs of life.

"Hand me an incisor; I want to make an incision," a surgeon might say to his nurse. Or "Give me a thorn;

Advance in instruments

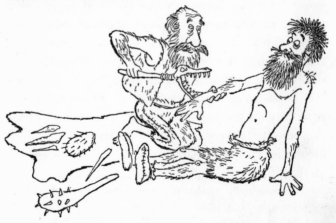

I want to see whether the fellow is really unconscious."

The first saws, we are told, were made of stone and bone, "obviously imitated from the teeth of animals." Why the Neolithic surgeon didn't make saws out of real teeth instead of imitation teeth, thus saving himself a lot of work, we shall never know. Our source goes on to say, "With these Holländer has performed amputations in six or seven minutes." It is hoped that Holländer got permission in writing from the patient or his next of kin before starting to saw with this primitive instrument. Otherwise he may have wound up with a malpractice suit on his hands.[1]

Skeletal remains indicate that one of the most frequent diseases of prehistoric man was arthritis. This resulted from contact with the damp walls and damp ground of caves, where these damp fools lived. Another theory is that they were forever stooping so as not to hit their heads, and this posture got to be a habit.

Whether the common cold was also prevalent cannot be discovered by examination of skeletons. However, we hazard a guess that it was, and that prehistoric medical researchers were already growing impatient at not finding a cure.

[1] Considering his speed with imitation animal teeth, one wonders what Holländer's time was with a good bone saw.

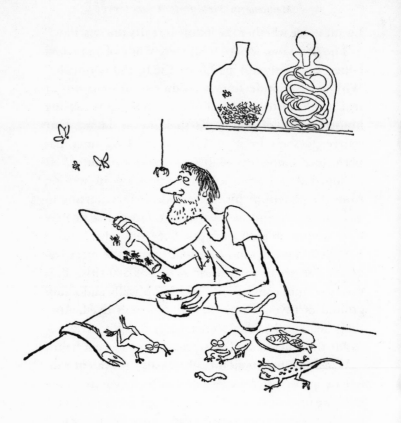

Chapter Two

PRIMITIVE

REMEDIES

It is not known precisely what remedies were used by prehistoric man, which is perhaps just as well. One curious cure, however, may be noted in connection with the trepanning mentioned above. It seems that these early people used the little round leftover pieces of skull to make amulets, which were supposed to ward off illness and are thought to be the origin of the modern charm bracelet.[1] While they were still fresh, they tended to ward off not only illness but anyone easily nauseated.

Otherwise we can only conjecture what remedies

[1] Digging pieces out of the skull may also have originated skulduggery.

were used in earliest times. If they were anything like those still in use by primitive peoples, they included the dried skin of a toad, to cure dropsy, and a beetle in a bottle for whooping cough.[1] Or the poor soul afflicted with malaria might wear a spider hung around his neck in a nutshell. Whether or not this did any good, getting a spider into a nutshell, and getting him to stay in, required so much concentration that the patient generally forgot what ailed him.

"That's it, in a nutshell," he would say tersely when the spider was safely inside.

Toads, beetles, and spiders were in great demand by the early equivalent of pharmaceutical houses. So were nutshells, which served the purpose very nicely until the invention of the capsule.

One of the most interesting early remedies was that used to reduce fever. First the patient's nails were clipped and the clippings were put in a little bag.[2] Then the bag full of nail clippings was hung around the neck of a live eel, which was placed in a tub of water. As the eel sickened, perhaps at the indignity of wearing a lavalier made of a complete stranger's nail

---

[1] There is something curative, or at least catchy, about "beetle in a bottle," said over and over. At any rate, while you are saying it you can't cough.

[2] For a mild fever, the fingernails were sufficient. But if the patient's temperature got up around 104°, it was a good idea to toss in the toenails also.

clippings, the patient felt better. By the time the eel died, the patient was completely well. Why this worked, no one could explain, but as the word got around among eels, they became harder and harder to catch.

Reference to things hung around the neck leads naturally enough to the necromancer and the use of magic in early medicine. When a patient was sick to his stomach, it did not occur to anyone that this might be the result of a diet of spoiled meat. Obviously an evil spirit or demon had got into him. Thus it was that the doctor, instead of sticking his finger down the patient's throat and encouraging him to get rid of the stuff, chanted magic words to expel the demon.[1] This was called "exorcising," and it was quite usual for a doctor to look at a patient and say, "What you need is more exorcise."

In early medicine much use was made of the "sympathy cure." In this, treatment was applied not to the patient but to what had hurt the patient. Thus when a rock fell on someone's head, the rock was covered with salve and bandaged. When sufficient time had passed, the bandages were removed from the rock, and everyone was gratified to find it as good as new.

"Not even a scar," the doctor would say smugly, after close examination.

---

[1] Perhaps something like "Yeah! yeah! yeah!"

Unfortunately, as medicine progressed and doctors became more sophisticated, they insisted on treating the patient himself. In the old days a patient who had been sliced open by a sword was spared the pain of being stitched up, while the sword was put to bed. But now the doctor went to work directly on the patient.

"Please, doctor," the patient protested, "while you are fiddling with me the sword is rusting. First things first, you know." Actually he was getting drowsy, as

Sympathy cure

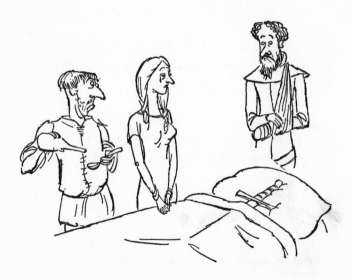

he bled to death, and was annoyed at being disturbed.

But enough of these newfangled methods. Let us leave this chapter with the haunting picture of an old-time doctor's bedside manner as he sat beside a bandaged rock or a bloody sword propped on a pillow, while the owner and his wife looked on anxiously.

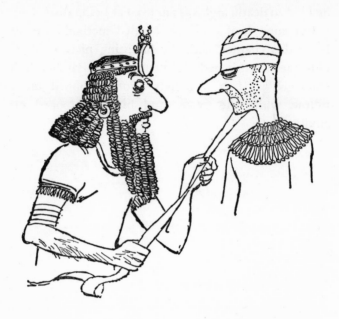

Chapter Three

THE BABYLONIANS
AND EGYPTIANS

The first code of medical ethics was drawn up by the Babylonian king, Hammurabi. According to the Code of Hammurabi, a doctor was to be paid so many shekels if, say, he opened an abscess and saved the eye of a patient. So far so good. But Hammurabi, who was always meddling, went a step further. "If he shall kill the patient or destroy the sight of the eye, his hands shall be cut off," said Hammurabi,[1] and this being before the AMA, there was no organized protest.

What we wonder is, who cut the doctor's hands off? Was it another doctor? And if he made a botch of it, were *his* hands cut off? When someone said to a doctor, "Hands off," warning him to keep out of

[1] Also referred to Big H and The Boss.

something, think of the scare it gave him. During the reign of Hammurabi, known as the Era of Amputation, young men were understandably reluctant to go into the medical profession.[1]

According to Herodotus, the Babylonians had another curious custom in the practice of medicine. The sick were brought out to the market place, and people passing by were expected to inquire about their disease. If a passer-by had had the same symptoms, he was to tell what treatment he had used. The market place was so full of the sick and those prescribing to them that it was hard to buy a head of cabbage. For those who liked to tell about their ailments and operations,[2] this was the Golden Age.

With the Egyptians, it became possible to read about medicine, thanks to medical tablets. These were not pills, as might be supposed, but clay bricks on which there was writing. Tablets in turn gave way to papyri, and papyrus prescriptions were much easier than clay bricks for patients to carry to the druggist. But doctors still did not make it too easy. So that the patient could make nothing of the prescription if he should peek, the doctor wrote in hieroglyphics.

[1] If it was a slave who lost his life as the result of an unsuccessful operation, the doctor had it somewhat easier. He had only to give the master another slave. And slaves, after all, were easier to replace than hands. Eventually, of course, slaves were replaced by hired hands.

[2] Roughly 99 per cent of the population.

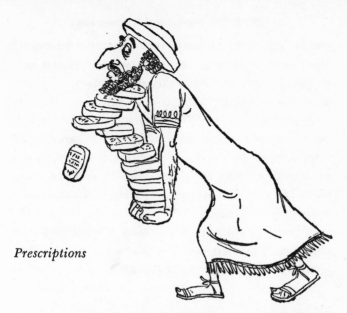

Prescriptions

About 4000 B.C., Egyptians began to use some sort of calendar. Previously it had been difficult to make an appointment with a doctor. What good did it do for the doctor to say, after thumbing through his appointment book, "I think I can see you on October 23rd," when neither he nor the patient had any idea when October 23rd was?

Medicine in ancient Egypt was presided over by various gods. Thoth, for instance, an ibis-headed god with a lisp, was the author of treatises on medicine.[1] The hawk-headed Horus, the god of health, lost an eye in a fight with Set, the demon of evil,[2] but

[1] A god-written treatise was as common those days as a ghost-written one is today.

[2] To lose to Set was considered a setback.

got it back miraculously. (How else?) The eye of
Horus was later made into the symbol ℞, on prescriptions, thus leading to the popular song, "The eye
of Horus is upon you." Finally there was Imhotep,
who started out as a human being and by some is
considered the first known physician, antedating
Hippocrates. This claim is muddied, however, by his
eventually coming to be worshipped as a god. Any
physician who is worshipped by his patients can be
grateful to Imhotep.

A study of mummies has proved enlightening with
regard to Egyptian medical practices. One medical
historian tells of "the great frequency of rheumatoid

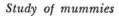

Study of mummies

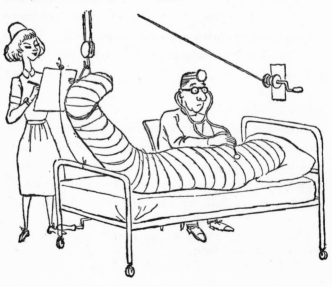

arthritis in Egyptian mummies, which was probably due to exposure during the inundations of the Nile." We had always thought mummies were beyond contracting illnesses, and shudder at the thought of all the things they are likely to pick up in the course of centuries.[1]

Of the many cures employed by Egyptians, one of the most interesting was a pomade for baldness, consisting of equal parts of fats of the lion, hippopotamus, crocodile, goose, serpent, and ibex. Any man who tracked down and killed all these creatures, extracted the fat, and smeared it on his head deserved to have hair, or at least an oily scalp.

Although it is not properly a part of medical history, a word should be said about Egyptian burial customs. Not only were people mummified but they were buried under enormously heavy pyramids, which were meant to hold them down. Anyone who was accidentally buried alive had to wait patiently for an archeological expedition.

[1] There is an article in the *British Medical Journal*, 1908, I, 732–737, about splints on mummies. If you think you might ever be called upon to put a splint on a mummy, you should read this.

Aesculapius

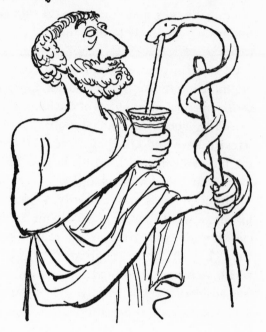

Chapter Four

AESCULAPIUS AND THE EARLY GREEKS

Babylonia and Egypt, we are told, "handed the torch of medical learning to the Greeks." Those who are familiar with the opening ceremony of the Olympic Games will be able to visualize this: a Babylonian doctor, with a torch held in his outstretched hand, running until he comes to another doctor who takes the torch and runs to another doctor who takes the torch and runs to another doctor, until at last the final doctor, torch in hand, staggers across the Greek border. The doctor is carried to the nearest hospital, suffering from exhaustion, dehydration, and third-degree burns on the arms and face, while the torch is used on a patient who had been waiting all this time to have a running sore [1] cauterized.

The Greeks gave a good deal of credit for medical

[1] Not to be confused with a running doctor.

advances to Apollo, the god of health, whose temple was at Delphi. People came from all over Greece for help. Apollo was not there himself, but he worked through an answering service. This was a priestess [1] who sat, chewing laurel leaves, by a cleft in the rock out of which came intoxicating fumes. People would tell her their symptoms and she would chew thoughtfully a few times, breathe deeply of the fumes, and give a prognosis. Actually the information came from Apollo, who was at the other end of the fumes, within easy reach of his Materia Medica.

Apollo taught the healing art to Chiron, a centaur who later became the god of surgery, and Chiron in turn taught Aesculapius. Since Chiron was half horse

[1] Or Sibyl, who hissed slightly, speaking in sibylants.

None too easy to teach

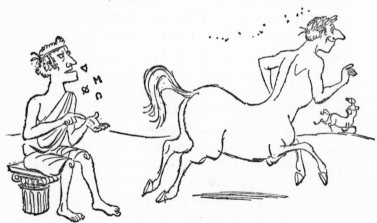

and half man, he was none too easy to teach, restlessly twitching his tail and often galloping off before the lesson was over, having spied an attractive filly.

As for Aesculapius, he was Apollo's son by an earthmaiden, Coronis. According to Hesiod, Apollo one day surprised Coronis bathing. She was not only surprised but astonished that Apollo, a god, would look at her, a little old virgin, that way. Anyhow, she tried to cover her embarrassment, being unable to cover anything else, and soon was carrying Apollo's child.[1] Unfortunately, her father had promised her to her cousin Ischus, and her condition was, after a few months, pretty obvious. To make a long story short, Apollo shot Ischus with an arrow, Artemis did likewise to Coronis, and then Apollo, feeling sorry for Coronis on her funeral pyre, snatched his unborn son, Aesculapius, from his mother's womb in what was surely the first instance of a Caesarian section.

Eventually Aesculapius took over Apollo's practice at Delphi, performing many miraculous cures, helped by his daughters Hygeia and Panacea, not to mention Edema and Pyorrhea. He was also helped by a trained snake, or medical technican, who went along to do little things such as licking a patient's sores or, if the the patient could hold still, his eyelids.[2]

---

[1] And not in her arms.

[2] If you have never had your eyelids licked by a snake, and are not ticklish, try it. Some find it as relaxing as a foot rub by a podiatrist.

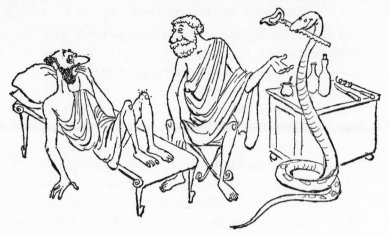

Medical assistant

As Aesculapius' name became known, he opened branches, known as Asklepieia, all over Greece. It was not ethical to advertise. Nor, as a matter of fact, was it necessary. His fame traveled to the remote coroners of Greece, and the sick hastened to the nearest Asklepieion for Aesculapius' patented cure. This was known as "incubation," or temple-sleep. The patient came to the temple (or incubator), went to sleep, and had a dream in which Aesculapius appeared and performed the treatment. After an incubation period of about eight hours, the patient awakened, feeling fine. It was a foolproof method, everyone being cured except an occasional insomniac.[1]

[1] Sometimes, instead of curing the patient while he slept, Aesculapius merely gave him a diagnosis, leaving treatment to his personal physician (priest) as a matter of professional courtesy.

One of Aesculapius' more spectacular cures, not widely achieved by physicians even today, was restoring the dead to life. What with curing his own patients and bringing back to life the patients of less successful doctors, Aesculapius was riding high. Then Pluto, the ruler of the Underworld, began to fear a shortage of population in his realm. So he appealed to Zeus,[1] who accommodatingly slew Aesculapius with a thunderbolt.

But don't feel sorry for Aesculapius. He was promoted from a demigod to a god, and lived happily ever after.[2]

---

[1] Pluto appealed to very few.

[2] As for his snake, it wound up (or around) a staff or wand, known as a caduceus.

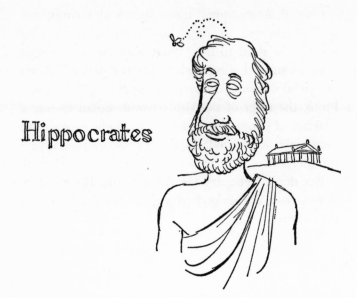

Hippocrates

Chapter Five

HIPPOCRATES AND THE LATER GREEKS

Before Hippocrates, medicine was in the hands of priests.[1] The priests thought diseases were caused by demons and angry gods, which still sounds pretty plausible. But Hippocrates thought sickness could be traced to natural causes, such as bad diet, lack of fresh air, too much carousing around, and falling off the top of the Parthenon.

"In truth we know little or nothing of Hippocrates," says one historian, preparatory to writing of him at length. It seems Hippocrates was born in 460 B.C. and lived until about 355 B.C., which, if our subtraction is correct, made him 105 years old at the time of his death. His ability to keep himself alive so

---

[1] In other words D.D.'s, not M.D.'s.

long must have been one reason he gained the confidence of his patients.[1]

But if Hippocrates lived a long time, think of the large plane tree, still pointed out as the one under whose shade he once taught his pupils. The age of this tree is estimated at around 2500 years, which shows that it knows a few things about health unknown to Hippocrates. But then, it stays out in the fresh air more than Hippocrates did, though it gets less exercise.

Hippocrates was born on the island of Cos, which explains the title of one of his many treatises, *The Cos and Effect of Disease*. Legend has it that he was once a librarian and was forced to flee when he burned some old medical books. Why he burned these books is not known. Did they disagree with his theories? An overworked librarian, was he tired of putting them back on the right shelf when they were misplaced by careless medical students? Was he cold, and out of kindling? The reader is left to his own conjectures.

Whether or not Hippocrates was forced to flee because of something he did as a librarian, there seems no doubt that he was an itinerant doctor. Since he had no office and for some reason declined to make house calls, he had to treat patients wherever

---

[1] A doctor suffering from a miserable head cold is always looked at a little skeptically when he holds out a handful of pills and says, "Take one of these three times a day and you'll feel better."

he found them—on the streets,[1] in the groves of Academe, or in the public bath. The bath was perhaps the most convenient, because patients wishing a thorough examination were already disrobed and ready to go. Anyhow, Hippocrates kept on the move, looking for a good plague. As Hippocrates' reputation grew, people came to him from all over Greece. This was flattering to Hippocrates but not to the patient's own doctor.

"What's this Hippocrates got that I haven't got?" the family physician would ask, with just a trace of a sneer. But there was no reply, because his former patients were too busy packing to go look for Hippoc-

[1] Accident victims.

Itinerant doctor

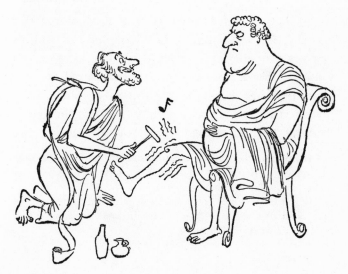

rates. There was a report he was last seen in Macedonia. Or was it Thrace? With Hippocrates wandering around looking for patients and patients wandering around looking for Hippocrates, there was a good deal of confusion.

Hippocrates based his medical practice on observation and reasoning, which have been the foundation of medicine ever since. For example, he would ask a patient to stick out his tongue, and he would look at it (observation). If it had a layer of whitish stuff on it, he would say to himself, "Aha, he had vanilla ice cream for dessert!" (reasoning). He was less interested in treatment than in diagnosis. Once he had figured out what was the matter with a patient and had told him, he felt he had discharged his responsibility. From then on, the patient could do the worrying. He was the one who was sick, wasn't he? [1]

An example of Hippocrates' method of practice was the time the King of Macedonia fell sick and his doctors thought he had phthisis.[2] Hippocrates was called in for a consultation and recognized at once that the King didn't have phthisis—he was off his rocker. Did Hippocrates attempt to cure the King? Did he tell the King, "Sire, you are nuts?" No,

[1] Hippocrates believed it was up to nature to do the healing. He referred his patients to nature the way GP's today refer their patients to specialists.

[2] If you have trouble pronouncing "phthisis," you might be interested to know that one of Hippocrates' biographers was named Tzetzes.

Hippocrates, who not only knew how to diagnose but when to keep his mouth shut, headed back to Athens as fast as he could go. Hippocrates has been called the Ideal Physician, and no wonder.

There are some fascinating legends about Hippocrates. One is that he never gave a thought to money. Another is that he admitted his errors. The reader should keep in mind that these are legends.

Ever since Hippocrates, graduating medical students take the Hippocratic oath, which starts out, "I swear." After they have been in practice a few years they learn how right Hippocrates was, and how much there is to swear about.

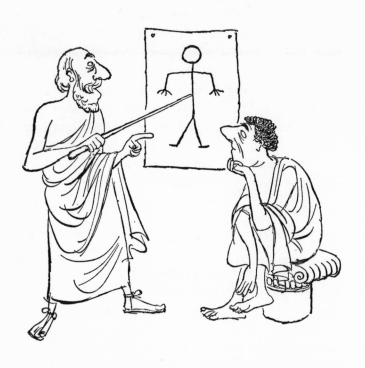

Chapter Six

TWO GREAT
ALEXANDRIANS

All histories of medicine mention two Alexandrian physicians, Herophilus and Erasistratus. It was Herophilus who named the duodenum, which until then medical men had only pointed at, saying, "That thing over there, next to the pylorus." He was also responsible for the depression in the occipital bone known as the *torcular Herophili*.[1] As if this were not enough, Herophilus counted the pulse, the rhythm of which he associated with music. "A-one, a-two, a-three," he chanted, closing his eyes, snapping his fingers, and smiling blissfully.

Erasistratus rejected the Greek idea of the humors. "I see nothing funny about them," he said stiffly. It was Erasistratus who not only distinguished the

[1] Responsible for the name of it, that is.

cerebrum from the cerebellum but also distinguished sensory from motor nerves. No wonder he is known as a distinguished physiologist.

What is most interesting about Herophilus and Erasistratus is the rumor that they practiced human vivisection. They are supposed to have done this with criminals, whom they removed from prison. Probably they removed them little by little, in a bag, so no one would notice.

Herophilus, by the way, is said to have been the first to practice public dissection of the human body.

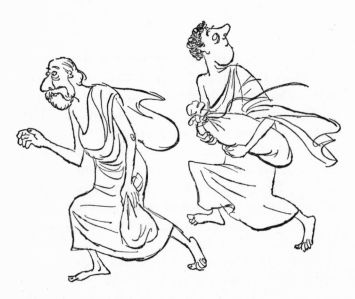

Removed them little by little

The first time, with everyone standing around gawking, that rhythmical *plunk! plunk!* was not the sound of a heartbeat but people fainting. It was clear that human dissection was not going to catch on as a spectator sport.

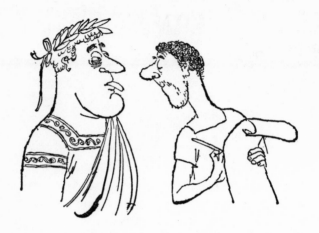

Chapter Seven

ROMAN

MEDICINE

Roman medicine made great contributions to sanitary engineering and public health. The Romans drained swamps, built aqueducts, constructed sewers, and killed off enough people in surrounding countries to keep cities from becoming overcrowded. Thanks to central heating, people kept warm, especially if they were near the center, and thanks to public baths, people kept clean. The baths were useful, too, for the study of anatomy.[1]

For a long time in Rome everyone was his own

---

[1] If an occasional virus was picked up in the public bath, this was more than offset by the juicy bits of gossip that could also be picked up.

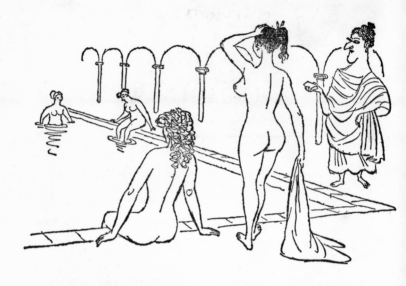

doctor—diagnosing himself, curing himself, and billing himself. It was the great Heal-It-Yourself Period. When the itinerant Greek physicians began to arrive (after a long walk), they were, naturally enough, down at the heel. Not being able to set up practice, they became slaves in wealthy Roman families. Still, they couldn't help dropping medicinal herbs and other goodies into the wine, and their masters were terribly afraid of being poisoned. The expression "Beware of Greeks bearing drugs" came in at this time, and it was not unusual for a high-borne [1] Roman to say, shrewdly, "Here, you take a swallow of this first." It is likely that the present distaste for medicine, especially by children who ask their parents to take a sip first, goes back to these worrisome times.

One of the itinerant physicians in Rome helped give medicine a good name.[2] This was Asclepiades,

[1] On a litter carried by four to six slaves, some of them perhaps M.D.'s.

[2] The name he gave it was Methodism, which seems a little odd, coming from a man who was not a Methodist.

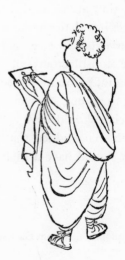

Study of anatomy

who had a theory that disease was caused by inconsiderate pores. If the pores were too contracted or too relaxed, there was trouble. They had to be just right. As a result of Asclepiades' teachings, doctors began to pore at pores for hours. Patients got better, but doctors suffered from eyestrain.

One of the earliest Roman medical men, though more of a writer than a practitioner, was Aurelius Cornelius Celsus, known as "the first important writer on medical history." [1] Celsus had a good deal to say about diet, which the Romans, busy gorging at orgies, paid no attention to whatsoever. In fact they were unable to hold Celsus' book, with both hands full of food. It was Celsus who mentioned the four cardinal signs of inflammation—*calor, rubor, tumor,* and *dolor*—and many wish he never had, because they are so hard to get out of your head once you have heard them.

Celsus wrote in elegant Latin, even when describing the tonsillectomy of that day. This involved reaching in, grabbing the tonsils with the fingers, and pulling them out. No wonder Celsus maintained that a physician should have a "strong and steady hand." He might have added that a patient facing a tonsillectomy should have a high threshold of pain.

[1] The quotation is from Garrison, not Celsus.

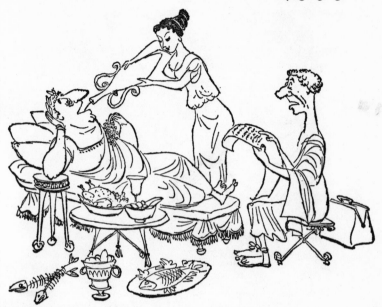

The most famous doctor in Rome was Galen.[1] He was also the cockiest. He had all the answers, and went around looking for questions. Galen flatly stated that he cured everyone, though there were those who hinted he may have swept a few patients under

[1] Galen's first name usually appears as "Cl." For centuries there had been a bitter controversy over whether the "Cl." stands for Claudius or Clarissimus. Those who do not wish to become involved are advised to refer to him simply as Galen.

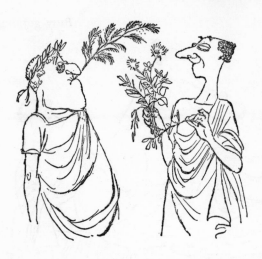

An herb for every disease

the rug. Herbs were his favorite cure. He had an herb
for every disease, and is even rumored to have fixed
a broken leg by using an asparagus stalk as a splint. In a
work called *De Simplicibus* he made everything
sound simple, refusing even to admit that there was
such a thing as a compound fracture.

He had some offbeat ideas about blood, which he
thought so full of Natural Spirit, Vital Spirit, and
Animal Spirit that there was no room for red and
white corpuscles. Nevertheless, everyone took him as
the final authority. If there was any question about a
medical matter, people said with a shrug, "Ask

Galen." Had he lived 1800 years later, he could have written a medical column and syndicated it in hundreds of newspapers.[1]

Galen made a big point of numerology, emphasizing the importance of five senses, four elements, four humors, two sexes, one head, etc. Everyone agrees with him about the importance of two sexes and shudders at the thought of there being even one more or one fewer.

At one point in his career Galen was the attending physician at gladiatorial contests, sitting on a bench by the coach. The gladiators afforded him considerable medical experience, but since his patients always recovered (see above), he had no corpses to dissect. His study of anatomy was therefore limited to cutting up apes and swine, which were not exactly like humans.[2]

An interesting medical theory is that the fall of Rome was caused by an epidemic of malaria. Most still prefer to believe, however, that it was overeating, with utter disregard of calories and cholesterol.[3]

---

[1] As it was, he wrote a vast amount. Probably the handiest edition is the 20-volume Greek and Latin text (Leipzig, 1821–33), which took twelve years to compile and takes almost as long to read.

[2] But close.

[3] Occasionally a Roman choked to death when a grape or an olive, dropped into his mouth by a slave, was slightly off target and lodged in the windpipe.

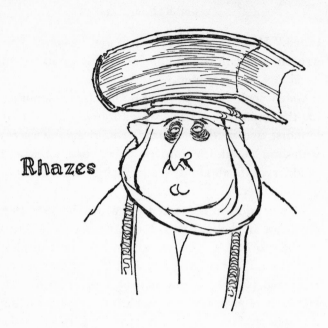

Rhazes

Chapter Eight

ARABIAN

MEDICINE

After the fall of Rome there was a period when most medical advances were made by the Arabs. The most remarkable Arab physician was Rhazes,[1] and the most remarkable thing about Rhazes was that one of his books, *Liber Continens,* weighed 22 pounds. Once he had a quarrel with the local ruler, who ordered him to be struck on the head with his own book (fortunately not *Liber Continens* but a smaller tome) until either his head or the book gave way. It was nip-and-tuck, and hard to tell whether those pieces falling to the ground were bits of parchment or bits of skull.[2] Rhazes became blind as a result of this, but refused

[1] Or, if you prefer, Abu Bekr Mohammed ibn Zakkariya, Ar-Razi.

[2] Rhazes also played the lute, but there is no evidence that he was ever beaten over the head with it.

an operation to restore his sight because he said he had seen enough already. Next time you break your glasses, you ought to meditate on Rhazes' remark before spending all that money for a new pair.

Smallpox and measles were very common among the Arabs, and in *On Smallpox and Measles,* one of the first monographs on a disease, Rhazes tried to help people figure out which it was they had. Of course those little red spots might merely be flea bites.[1] It could have been Rhazes who made the classic statement, subsequently translated into many languages: "Don't scratch!" [2]

And then there was Avicenna. A precocious youngster, he took up the study of medicine at sixteen, and at eighteen was a famous physician. By the time he was twenty-one he had written a twenty-volume medical encyclopedia. Young doctors of today, just completing their internship at twenty-six or twenty-seven, and with residency and military service yet ahead, should be ashamed of themselves.

It is appropriate that Avicenna, who was hotter than a pistol, should have written a work called *Canon.* In this he had the modest ambition of compiling *everything* known about medicine. A winebibber, Avicenna discovered wine as a dressing for wounds when he overturned a glass while attending a

[1] Not to be confused with phlebitis.

[2] For asthma, Rhazes prescribed two drachmas of dried and powdered fox lung, taken in the patient's drink. It may not have helped asthma, but it cut down drinking.

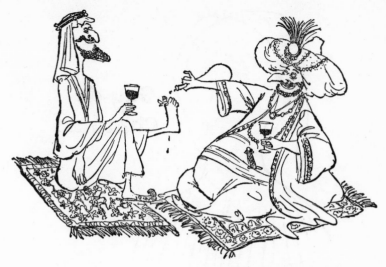

Dressing for wounds

patient. Wine, women, and song (not necessarily in that order) did him in while he was in the prime of life. In view of his early start, however, he had already had a full life.

The Arabs built great hospitals at Baghdad, Damascus, and Cairo. At one hospital fifty speakers recited the Koran day and night, and patients could hardly wait to get back to the peace and quiet of home. Nothing equaled this as a means of cutting down the stay of in-patients until someone thought of waking them every few minutes through the night to take their temperature or give them an enema.[1]

[1] Despite what you may have read, Arabian nights were no fun—not if you were a patient in the Baghdad hospital.

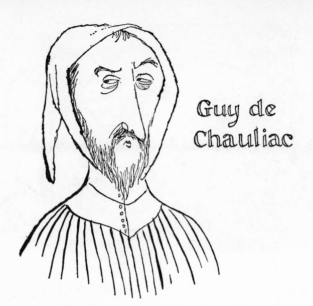

Guy de
Chauliac

Chapter Nine

MEDICINE IN
THE MIDDLE AGES

Medicine took an unexpected turn in the Middle Ages, when it became affiliated with astrology. No one would swallow a pill without first checking to see whether the stars were in a favorable position, and on a cloudy night this could be difficult. The horoscope was used more than the microscope.[1]

A good deal of dependence was also put on magic, of which there were two kinds: black magic and white magic. Black magic was powerful stuff, sold under the counter, and you had to know a magician to get it.

During the Middle Ages medicine came under the control of the Church, and monks picked up some extra money moonlighting as doctors. If a monk was

[1] In this respect, medicine was looking up.

called out on a case in the middle of the night, he was on his way in a jiffy, since he had only to throw on his bathrobe and he was fully dressed.[1]

In connection with the influence of the Church on medicine, it should be noted that saints became associated with the healing of various diseases. If you had a sore throat, for example, you prayed to Saint

Moonlighting

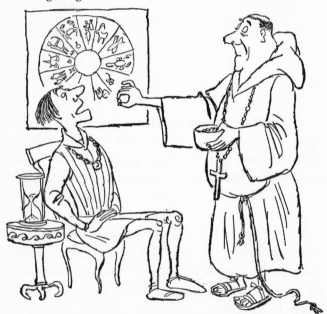

[1] Though no Pope is known to have become a physician, one physician became a Pope. This was Petrus Hispanus, who became Pope John XXI. It might have been better had he remained a physician, since he was killed when the ceiling of his palace fell on him.

Blaise. For insanity it was Saint Dymphna.[1] For hemorrhoids it was Saint Fiacre. The saints were inclined to be specialists rather than GP's.

This was a great time for the quack. The original quack was probably a veterinary surgeon who specialized on the vocal cords of ducks. As time went on, the quack broadened his sphere to human beings and to other parts of the body. Eventually a quack became any medical practitioner with whose methods you disagree.

Blood letting was a popular cure in the Middle Ages. The idea was to get rid of impurities in the blood by opening a vein or (if in a hurry) an artery and letting the patient almost bleed to death. Much of the blood letting was accomplished by barbers, some of whom were very accomplished. There was also considerable therapeutic blood letting in tournaments, when knights with lances, tilting full tilt, could lance a good deal more than a boil.

With reference to barbers as blood letters,[2] it should be remarked that they also performed minor surgery, in which case they tilted the barber chair all the way back, wrapped some especially hot cloths over the patient's face to distract him from other pain, and stropped their scalpels to a fine edge. During surgery, a barber kept his patient's mind off the cutting by

[1] This is a name that lingers with you, especially if you are slightly insane.

[2] After a particularly busy day, a barber might remark to his colleague at the next chair, "A red-letter day, wasn't it?"

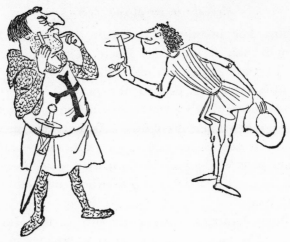

Minor surgery

telling him the latest scuttlebutt of the court, the odds on Saturday's big tournament between the Christians and Pagans, and what ought to be done about the Black Death. After surgery he usually asked, "Would you like a scalp massage, with tonic?" and "How about a manicure?" [1]

Surgery was in a low state during the Middle Ages. The physician looked down on the surgeon, the surgeon looked down on the barber, and the barber, standing by the barber chair, looked down on the patient.

One reason surgery was in low regard was that a surgeon was severely dealt with if his patient failed to come through an operation. According to one medical

[1] In addition to performing minor surgery, the medieval barber "gave enemas, picked lint, and extracted teeth." The barber shop was a busy place, and anyone waiting for a chair could keep amused without reading girlie magazines.

historian, "In 1337, a strolling eye surgeon [1] was thrown into the Oder because he failed to cure John of Bohemia of his blindness." Surgeons were in bad Oder indeed.

The most difficult cases were usually handled by itinerant surgeons, who got out of town while the patient was still on the critical list.

From the standpoint of the patient, surgery may have been downgraded because of the anesthesia then in use. This was the so-called "soporific sponge." It wasn't its being steeped in a mixture of opium, hyoscyamus, mulberry juice, lettuce, hemlock, and mandragora that disturbed the patient. It was his having to swallow it, sponge and all. "Come now," the anesthetist would say, using an expression later taken over by dentists, "open wide." [2]

This was when knighthood was in flower. Knights in full armor were something of a problem when they came into a doctor's office for an examination. For one thing, they were noisy, clanking around in the waiting room trying to find an illuminated manuscript they hadn't already read. For another, it was hopeless to try to feel a pulse through a metal sleeve and rather silly to ask a grown man to stick out his tongue through a visor. But getting a knight to disrobe was no fun either, since he couldn't do it himself, and a nurse usually wasn't strong enough to lift

[1] He should have run.

[2] See also the expression "Throw in the sponge," which in those days was "Throw up the sponge."

some of the larger pieces of metal. This meant the doctor had to lend a hand, when his waiting room was filling up and there were house calls to make.

Often a knight who had been fighting a fire-breathing dragon would come in with third-degree burns. What pained him was not so much the burns as their being on his back, thus giving people the impression that he had been running away, which was correct. Or a fire-breathing dragon might come in and ask for something for his breath.

Never a dull moment for the medieval physician. And no telling who, out in that crowded waiting room, was coming down with the plague.

Disrobing

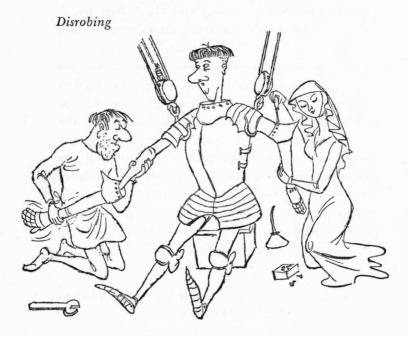

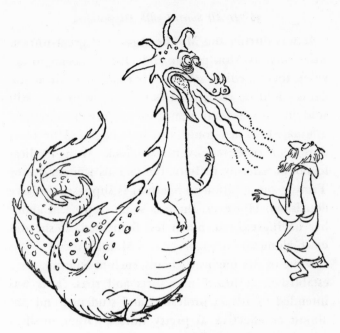

Something for his breath

Sorcery and superstition played a large part in medieval medicine. To remove a bone from the throat, for example, the physician recited a long incantation, completely without meaning,[1] all the while moaning and swaying rhythmically. At the end of the incantation he would shout, "Bone come up or bone go down." What was shrewd about this was giving the bone a choice. It showed, even in those early times, a knowledge of psychology.

[1] Sounding for all the world like the commencement address at a medical school.

It was during the Middle Ages that great universities such as Montpellier and Oxford began to develop their medical schools. Henceforth medical students could be recognized as the ones who were still studying for several years after everyone else had graduated.[1] They could also be recognized by their drawn, or sometimes overdrawn, look. At the medical school of Salerno, in Italy, the famous woman doctor Trotula (no relation to Spatula) is supposed to have flourished. However, there is some skepticism about her having existed, much less flourished. If she did exist, along about 1050, she was Middle Aged.[2]

Some of the medical schools, such as Salerno, were established at healthful resorts and spas. This was intended to attract professors and students, and was almost as effective as pretty nurses. Other medical schools were founded in great population centers such as Paris, where there were plenty of diseased people to practice on.

It was at Salerno that the title "Doctor" was first applied to a graduate of a medical school. This was later shortened to "Doc."

One of the great scholars of the Middle Ages was Roger Bacon, who taught at Oxford and Paris, where he went around under the pseudonym of Doctor

[1] Sometimes theological students were even slower graduating, being in the midst of an argument and not noticing it was June.

[2] She was sometimes called Dame Trot, because of her peculiar way of walking. The Russian form of this is Trotsky.

Mirabilis. Whether or not he was a physician, he was a physicist, philologist, mathematician, philosopher, chemist, and geographer. Though also a writer, he is not to be confused with the author of Shakespeare's plays. He was always experimenting, and has been credited with inventing the telescope, the microscope, the diving bell, gunpowder, spectacles, locomotives, and airplanes. Had he lived a few years longer, he might have thought of the telephone, radio, television, and penicillin.

Late in life Bacon, according to his biographer, "incurred the displeasure of the Church." And no wonder, since he published a book in which he attacked the ignorance and vices of the clergy, and these gentlemen could, after all, be sensitive about such things. Anyhow, he was given fourteen years in prison to think it over. These fourteen years, besides another period of ten years when he was under house arrest and prohibited from writing anything for publication, cut down his literary output. Some, who are familiar with the scope and magnitude of Bacon's writings, think he was put away not so much because he insulted the clergy as because of fear he would deplete the supply of ink, quill pens, and parchment in France and England.[1]

Mention should also be made of that famous medieval surgeon, Guy de Chauliac, who studied medicine

---

[1] One book Bacon failed to finish, and from its title it sounds like a potential best seller, is *Liber Sex Scientiarum*. In it Bacon planned to embrace everything.

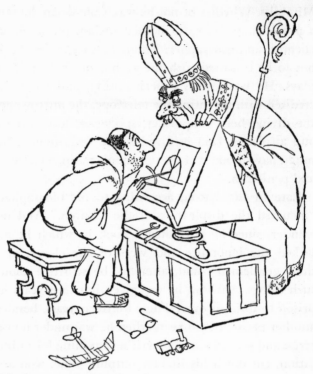

Displeasure of the Church

at Toulouse, Montpellier, Paris, and Bologna—a record that should encourage students who don't make it the first time. He was immensely learned, especially about medical schools. The most memorable thing about Guy is his having been probably the first to employ traction in the treatment of a fracture. Anyone with a broken thigh who has been ingeniously trussed up with ropes, pulleys, and weights until he looks like a spider weaving a web should thank Guy de Chauliac and not Rube Goldberg.

By the end of the Middle Ages things looked pretty bad for medicine, though perhaps not as black as during the Dark Ages. It is true that spectacles were invented.[1] And artificial limbs came into use, after a period of experimenting with the limbs of trees. Moreover, rules were developed for medical etiquette, including the requirement that the doctor should approach the bedside "with humble mien" and "should not diminish his professional status by ogling the patient's wife, daughter, or maid-servants." These were unquestioned improvements.

On the other hand (or wherever), the testicles were often removed, in an operation for hernia, simply because they got in the way. And urine specimens were delivered to the physician by messenger, to facilitate examination in absentia, the patient himself trying to remain aloof from the whole business.[2] As late as the fourteenth century the patient being treated for epilepsy was required to write the words Melchior, Jasper, and Balthazar with blood from his little finger and wear for a month a sheet of paper bearing these words. Whether the patient wore anything else our source does not disclose.

Obviously there was still room for improvement in the practice of medicine, and most patients could hardly wait for the Renaissance.

[1] If you are having trouble with your eyes, are interested in the history of spectacles, and can read German, see (as well as you can) R. Greeff, *Die Erfindung der Augengläser,* Berlin, 1921.

[2] Especially (see above) if he thought a hernia operation might be indicated.

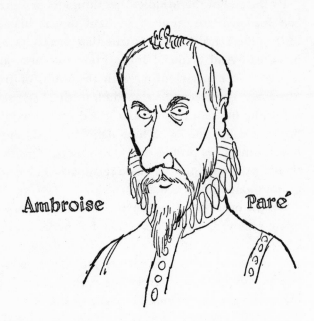

Ambroise Paré

Chapter Ten

THE

RENAISSANCE

On May 29, 1453, Constantinople fell and the Renaissance began. Horizons widened. Thought became free. People's eyes were opened. Everyone took a critical attitude, and medical men said some pretty sharp things about old-fashioned Galen. Galen, poor fellow, was unable to defend himself, having died in 201 A.D.

Two important inventions were gunpowder and printing. Gunpowder, which made prince and peasant equal, if they were both armed, was known as the great leveler. It leveled hundreds of thousands, of all classes, and produced the hole man of the Renaissance. Until the invention of gunpowder, no one knew how to remove a bullet or treat a powder burn. As for printing, this led inevitably to the publication of medical magazines, which piled up unread in the doctor's office and gave him a guilt complex. Or, if he took the time to read all the articles in his field so that he could practice more effectively, he had to give up his practice.[1]

Thanks also to printing, manuscripts were replaced by printed medical books, complete with plates, tables, and typographical errors. The first medical work printed in England was a little tract entitled *A Passing Gode Lityll Boke Necessarye and Behovefull Against the Pestilence*. The advice it contained was somewhat better than the spelling.

Renaissance artists like Michelangelo and Leonardo da Vinci, eager to understand anatomy, practiced dissection, sometimes working with a brush in one hand and a scalpel in the other. Leonardo, in fact, discovered the maxillary sinus and other parts of the body that seldom show up in his paintings. Most art lovers who admire the subtle smile of his Mona Lisa are unaware that this versatile artist also left us some beautiful drawings of the viscera.

Everyone knows that in this great era of discovery Columbus discovered the New World. Not so many know that Columbus discovered pulmonary circulation. The discoverer of pulmonary circulation was Realdus Columbus, who was born four years after Christopher died.[2]

[1] Doctors who wrote for medical journals exchanged articles (called reprints) with other doctors who wrote for medical journals, each thinking the other got the better of the exchange.

[2] What do *you* celebrate on Columbus Day?

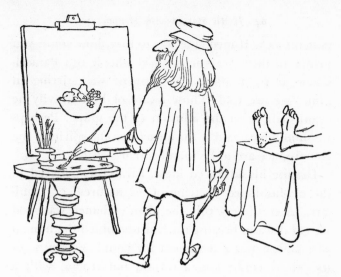

Leonardo

The spirit of the Renaissance is to be found in Paracelsus, a quarrelsome Swiss physician whose middle name was Bombastus.[1] Paracelsus wandered all over Europe carrying a staff, not to help himself walk but to defend himself. Everywhere he went he made enemies. For one thing, he wrote in German instead of Latin, and scholars who had spent years learning Latin resented this. Furthermore, he tended to oversimplify. He declared that man is composed of three elements—sulphur, mercury, and salt—and too much or too little of any one of these is what makes a person sick. There were, he maintained, only three diseases and three cures. The very idea made Paracelsus' op-

[1] It really was.

ponents sick. If medicine was so easy, how could you justify all those years in medical school? But Paracelsus went right ahead. "A ferment was stirring in him," we are told. Those aware of how heavily he drank will catch the allusion to the grape. Perhaps we should have said at the outset that the spirits of the Renaissance are to be found in Paracelsus.

Despite his advanced ideas, Paracelsus believed in the old-fashioned doctrine of "signatures" or "similars." According to this, the plant cyclamen was good for ear diseases because the leaf resembled the human ear; saffron was a treatment for jaundice because of its yellow color; and a certain mushroom, with a phallic shape, was prescribed for impotence. What stumped Paracelsus, though, was trying to find a plant that had the shape and color of the common cold.

The greatest anatomist of the Renaissance was Andreas Vesalius, who was born in Brussels but did much of his work in Padua. As a boy, he cut up dogs, cats, mice, rats, and moles. When animals saw him coming, they ran for their lives. He could hardly wait to get at human beings, and the way he looked at people made them uneasy.

When he was in medical school, Vesalius was the envy of his fellow students. He had his own skeleton! [1] To get hold of it, he did what any medical student would have done if he had had the opportunity: he stole the body of a criminal from the gallows. How he

[1] That is to say, he possessed the skeleton of someone else.

got it home we do not know, but it must have been an exciting evening.

Unlike Galen, who dissected animals, Vesalius made a firsthand [1] study of the human body. Galen had assumed that the anatomy of animals and humans was the same, but Vesalius discovered all kinds of subtle differences between, say, a man and a dog, which had escaped Galen completely.

Vesalius' eagerness to dissect the human body may have been his undoing. The story is told that he was in Madrid, starting to perform a post-mortem examination, when the corpse began to show signs of life. Many thought Vesalius should have waited just a few minutes longer. Anyhow, he excused himself, say-

[1] First one hand and then the other, and so on.

Subtle differences

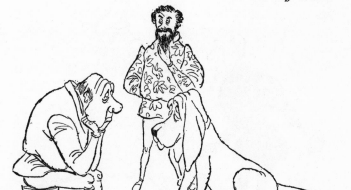

ing he had to go to the Holy Land. He never came back.

Had it not been for Fallopius (who succeeded Vesalius at Padua) and Eustachius (who taught anatomy at Rome), who can guess what names would have been given to the Fallopian tube and the Eustachian tube? [1]

Mention should be made of that great Frenchman, Ambroise Paré, known as the Father of Modern Sur-

---

[1] In London when a doctor says he is going to "take the tube," there is no telling whether he intends to go by Underground or to operate.

Paré attended four kings

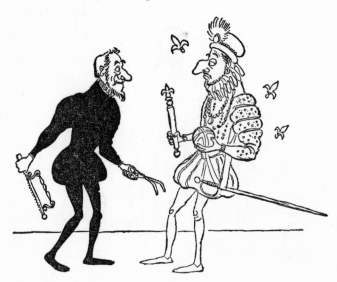

gery.[1] In his lifetime France was almost constantly at war—against Italy, Germany, and England, and, in a civil war, against France. Paré joined the army as a surgeon, expecting to get a little experience with gunshot wounds before settling down to practice in Paris and making a good thing out of duels and crimes of passion. What with one war and another, however, he stayed in the army for thirty years.

[1] Though he was much in Germany and Italy, Paré kept his French accent. It is an acute accent, over the *e*. With all the cutting he did, the name Pare, without the accent, would have been more appropriate.

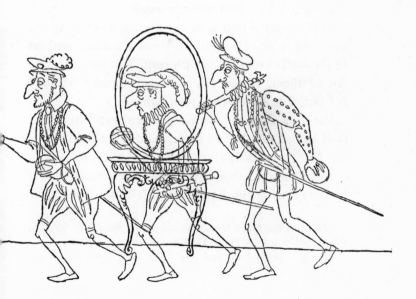

Paré is known to have been humane and kindly. Cutting into a patient hurt him more than it did the patient, Paré not being anesthetized. The common practice was to pour boiling oil into gunshot wounds, to cauterize them. Wounded soldiers, who hadn't much minded being shot, yelled bloody murder while this was going on. Paré, who was tenderhearted, could hardly stand to hear this screaming, yet he went right on pouring. In one battle so many soldiers had gunshot wounds that he ran out of boiling oil. He was forced to take care of the remaining soldiers by smearing on a little salve.[1] To his great astonishment, the soldiers with the salve on their wounds came out better than those with the boiling oil. "Wonderful!" exclaimed kindhearted Paré. "Now I won't have to listen to all that horrible screaming."

Paré attended four Kings of France, some of whom were sickening. He outlived them all, and members of the court viewed this with suspicion. However the last of them, Henry III, was assassinated, and Paré got out of this one with clean hands.[2]

Paré's favorite expression was "I dressed him, and God healed him." Paré preferred doing things alone, but in a partnership like this he couldn't lose.

Finally a word about the Medici, the greatest family in Italy during the Renaissance. It is not quite clear

[1] Made of the fat of freshly boiled puppy dogs. The S.P.C.A. was unimpressed by Paré's kindness to people.

[2] He had washed up and was ready to operate, but it was too late.

whether Medicine was named after the Medici or the Medici were named after Medicine.[1] Mostly the Medici were patrons of artists and writers rather than doctors, which may explain why they died out in 1743, surrounded by books and paintings but in bad shape physically.

[1] Sir Thomas Browne's *Religio Medici*, by the way, has nothing to do with the religion of the Medici.

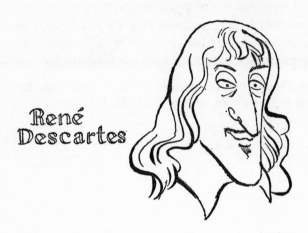

René
Descartes

Chapter Eleven

MEDICINE IN THE SEVENTEENTH CENTURY

Many consider the seventeeth century the Golden Age of medicine. Doctors knew much more than previously, but patients still didn't know enough to challenge their every statement. Gold, which in the Middle Ages was taken by patients to improve their health, now was taken by doctors to improve their financial status.

This was also an age of inquiry. Doctors were always asking each other, "What's new?" and "Heard any good medical stories lately?" [1] Patients asked, "Will I live?" and "How much?"

---

[1] By good they meant bad, the kind that makes doctors look around to see whether any nurses are within earshot.

The philosophers pointed the way. One of these was Francis Bacon, who as Lord Verulam sounded like the trade name for a high-class drug. He helped medicine by stressing experiment and the inductive method of reasoning, based upon experience. At the same time, he made it harder for people who henceforth had to remember which is inductive and which is deductive.[1]

Bacon annoyed nutritionists, dentists, and librarians when he said, in one of his essays, "Some books are to be tasted, others to be swallowed, and some few to be chewed and digested." They disagreed most violently with Bacon in their belief that all books, and not just a few, should be chewed before being swallowed. Always the experimenter, Bacon became ill and died as a result of trying to stuff a chicken with snow. He should have used bread crumbs, chopped onion, and seasoning.

Another important philosopher was René Descartes. He did an interesting thing. He tried to empty his mind of everything he had learned and start all over. There were a few days, before his mind started to fill up again, when he was in bad shape mentally. Descartes believed in thinking. "I think, therefore

---

[1] One way to remember is to think of the word "pig," the letters of which stand for particular-inductive-general. Thus the inductive method is to go from particulars to the general. The deductive method is the opposite, which you can remember by keeping in mind the word "gdp."

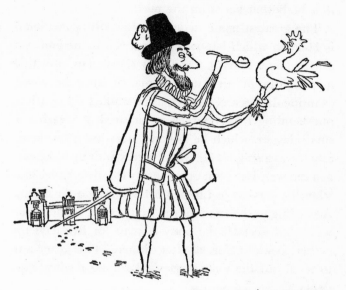

Always the experimenter

I am," he said. But at times of uncertainty he more cautiously said, "I think I think, therefore I think I am, I think." All this greatly encouraged experimental physicians, some of whom even experimented with thinking. Why not give it a try?

Descartes, by the way, was interested in physiology, and thought he had located the soul—in the pineal gland. Apparently the soul of the average person isn't very large, since the pineal gland is about the size of a pea.[1] But a little soul goes a long way, especially in a body that keeps on the move.

The greatest name in seventeeth-century medicine is Harvey, which happens to be a last name and not a first name. Harvey was a very short man, and this helped him in his study of plants, since he could examine daisies and pansies, as he walked along, without bending over. Harvey is pictured as wearing a small dagger, which he fingered nervously, but actually it was a scalpel. He could hardly wait until he got at a cadaver. His great opportunity for dissection came when he was made Lumleian Lecturer on Anatomy. According to the terms of the lectureship, the lecturer was "to dissect all the body of man for five days together, as well before as after dinner." This latter was to weed out the weak-stomached among medical students.

Before Harvey, the liver was thought to be the central motive force of the blood, and blood was thought to move to-and-fro. Harvey became convinced that instead of going to-and-fro, blood goes around and around. This is very economical, since a little blood (see the soul, above) goes a long way, and people should be a lot more grateful than they are. He also thought the heart clenched and unclenched like a fist, though not mad about a thing. When Harvey published his findings, many refused to believe

[1] Try telling someone, "You've got a soul about the size of a pea," and see what it gets you.

him, and his practice fell off. Patients didn't want to go to a physician who had such crazy ideas. He might put a tourniquet around their neck to see whether it made them red in the face. But Harvey lived to see his ideas accepted. Living to be almost eighty helped.

It was Harvey who conducted the post-mortem examination of Thomas Parr, who died at the age of 153 years. Parr had enjoyed perfect health all his life and had married twice, first at the age of 88 and again at 120. Harvey found that Parr's death was due to pleuropneumonia, though there were those who thought it might have been something else, such as old age.

Although patients regarded Harvey as an extraordinary physician, he was only Physician-in-Ordinary to King Charles I. Harvey served the King well, but was unable to help him when that unlucky monarch had his head cut off. There was too much loss of blood.[1] Earlier, Harvey had accompanied the King to a battle, and was sitting there reading a book and waiting for someone to get shot when bullets began to come close. With not a little annoyance, he closed his book and moved out of the line of fire. While others lost their lives, he lost his place.[2]

[1] In his classic work on the circulation of the blood, Harvey compared the heart to the King, the center of strength and power. Some say the King, to whom Harvey dedicated the book, was pleased.

[2] Medical man that he was, he may have been somewhere in the appendix.

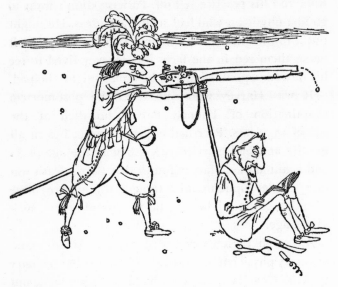

Waiting for someone to be shot

One of the things that helped medical research at this time was invention of the microscope. Though the first to use a microscope to study the causes of disease may have been Kircher, the most important name in this field, and the hardest to spell, was Leeuwenhoek. Leeuwenhoek was a Dutch merchant who, instead of growing tulips or sticking his finger in a hole in the dike, spent his spare time fooling around with microscopes. He had them all over the house—247 of them, to be exact. When he came home from work, his wife would throw up her hands and cry, "What? Another one?" Not only did he discover red corpuscles, but he was the first to see and describe bacteria. It is not known what he said when he had his first look, probably "Ugh!" One day, examining under a microscope the white film that collected on his teeth, he saw "little animals, more numerous than all the people in the Netherlands, and moving about in the most delightful manner." [1] From then on, nothing was too disgusting for this inquisitive Dutchman.

[1] How Leeuwenhoek got the microscope into his mouth and managed to look through it remains a mystery.

Fooling around with microscopes

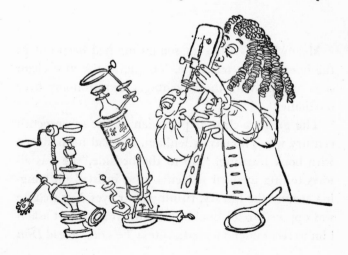

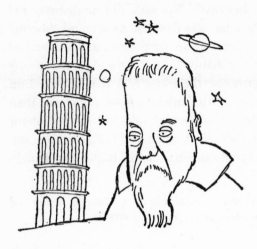

Galileo

Meanwhile Galileo for some time had been out in the open with a telescope, looking at the nice clean stars and proving the advantages of astronomy over medicine.

The greatest clinical physician of the seventeenth century was Thomas Sydenham. He had no patience with book learning. "Go to the bedside," he was always telling medical students, who insisted on hanging around the library, ruining their eyes. Not that he was opposed to all books. Once when a student asked him to recommend a medical text, he said, "Read *Don*

Quixote." He probably thought the part where Don Quixote tilts at windmills would provide some hints about how to lance boils on a patient who won't sit still.

Though Sydenham was at first regarded as an eccentric, he came to be admired by many. In fact there was one physician who, when lecturing to his medical students, raised his hat every time he said "Sydenham." It was a nice little gesture, but distracting.[1]

Some of the most vivid medical writing of the seventeenth century or any century is to be found in Sydenham's *A Treatise on the Gout.* As Sydenham describes it: "The pain becomes intense. Now it is a violent stretching and tearing of the ligaments, now it is a gnawing pain and now a pressure or tightening.... The night is spent in torture." One thing that helped him in writing about the gout was that he had it, and bad. This suggests that we would have better writing about diseases if doctors were sicker.

A disease that reached its height (in the lymphatic glands of the neck) at this time was a type of scrofula known as King's Evil. It was cured by the Royal Touch—in other words, being touched by the King. In a number of touching scenes, Charles II set an all-time record by touching 6,725 persons in a single

---

[1] Apparently doctors kept their hats on in the house in those days. In medical school they taught almost everything but manners.

year. His lifetime total was 92,107.[1] Some came from afar to be touched. In the mob milling around the King, many were trampled to death, thus being cured not only of King's Evil but of getting into a crowd.

On this happy note let us leave the seventeenth century.

---

[1] What fascinates us about these figures is who kept count of the touches. And whether there were any doubtful ones, or balks.

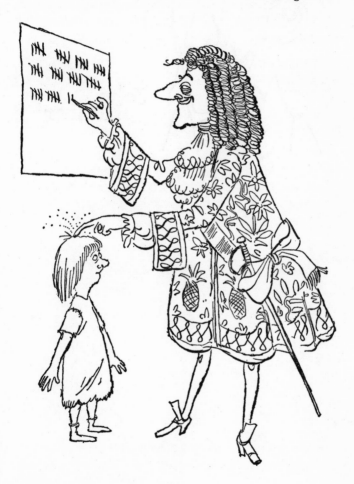

Touching scene

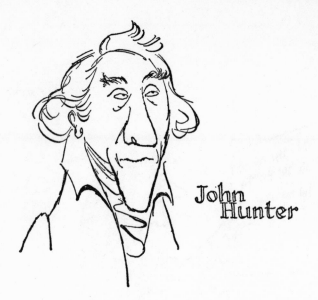

John
Hunter

Chapter Twelve

MEDICINE IN THE
EIGHTEENTH
CENTURY

In the eighteenth century doctors wore wigs, even when they had a good head of hair. In addition to wigs, they wore fancy breeches, a velvet coat with gilt buttons, buckled shoes,[1] and a three-cornered hat. They usually carried a cane with a gold top, the top containing smelling salts which they could sniff when near a patient who hadn't bathed for several months. The average doctor was a dandy.[2] Yet, fancily though he tricked himself out, he dressed wounds quite simply.

[1] Doctors themselves often buckled, after a hard day in such a costume.

[2] But not necessarily a dandy doctor.

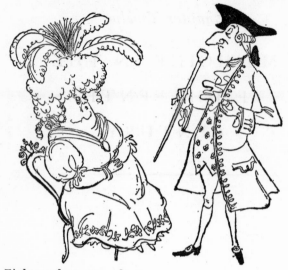

Eighteenth-century doctor

One of the great medical men of the century was Linnaeus, a Swedish botanist and physician. He studied medicine in order to win the daughter of a wealthy practitioner, who refused his consent to the marriage unless the prospective son-in-law would become a doctor.

"Anything but that," Linnaeus begged, but the girl's father was adamant. He wanted Linnaeus to join him in medical practice so he could take a vacation without having to refer patients to someone outside the family and maybe lose them for good.

"You'd better do as he says, Lin," the girl said, lifting her skirt enough for him to catch a tantalizing glimpse of a pair of gorgeous ankles. Linnaeus, though he hated himself for it, gave in.

He was a great classifier. He classified everything: plants, animals, minerals, man. A tidy sort, he was not satisfied until everything was in a pigeonhole with a label on it. In his office if you looked under "P" until you found "Primate" and then looked under "Primate" until you came to *"Homo sapiens,"* you would find what you were looking for—"Man."

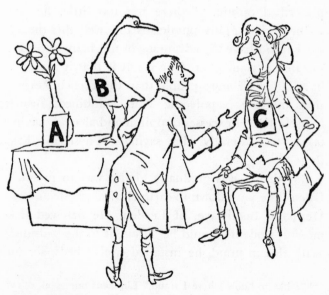

Great classifier

Or you could look under "M" until you found "Man" and then work your way back to "Primate." If you had plenty of time, you could do this for days.[1]

A specialty of Linnaeus' was the sex life of plants. While others did nothing more with flowers than sniff them or stick them into vases, he crept up close and looked at their stamens and pistils. But they weren't embarrassed. After all, he was an M.D.

There were many interesting medical theories in the eighteenth century. One of these was advanced by John Brown, whose Brunonian theory held that disease is the result of either too much or too little excitement in the body. If there was too much, he prescribed opium. If there was too little, he prescribed wine. Many physicians followed this theory, since it *did* have the advantage of not being too complicated to remember. One result is that it is said to have killed off more people than the French Revolution and the Napoleonic Wars combined. Brown himself died of excesses of opium and alcohol, having taken too literally the saying, "Physician, heal thyself."

But theory was gradually giving way to practice. One of the most down-to-earth clinical physicians was Hermann Boerhaave, of Leyden. He believed that medical students should be "brought to the bedside." With this in mind, he installed twelve beds, six for

[1] "I like to know where I stand," Linnaeus once said, drawing chalk marks around his feet.

men patients and six for women, and took his students with him on his rounds.

"Watch my bedside manner," he said to them, as they trailed along, notebooks in hand. The time he tripped on a bedpan and took a tumble, getting a good laugh and setting the patient at ease, they all jotted down: "Bedpan—trip—patient enjoys." Then they hurried over to help Boerhaave, who had fractured his right tibia.[1]

With his students clustered around, Boerhaave would lecture while he examined the patient, giving a detailed diagnosis and plan of treatment. The patient, meanwhile, learned all about himself. He felt pretty important, being the center of all that attention, until Boerhaave made some such remark as "This case, gentlemen, is hopeless."

There was quite an upsurge of medicine in Scotland at this time. Scottish physicians had something of an advantage because their burr was so thick their patients couldn't understand them. Thus, when a doctor prescribed a potion and it was the wrong thing, the patient didn't take it, and recovered. One of these Scotsmen was Alexander Wood, who was accompanied on his professional rounds by a tame raven and a sheep. Why he had these companions is not

---

[1] Of course Boerhaave had planned the whole thing. An experienced teacher, he knew how important it is to hold the students' attention.

known. Perhaps the raven went ahead to knock on the door.[1] The sheep, looking sheepish, was counted over and over by insomniacs, who found this better than barbiturates. Anyhow, Wood liked the companionship of his animals, and no doubt managed to take them off his income tax as a necessary expense. Wood, by the way, was the first person in Edinburgh to carry an umbrella. He was thought an eccentric until it rained.

One Scottish physician who was not first at anything nonetheless achieved a certain degree of fame

[1] Which was better than knocking on Wood.

Alexander Wood

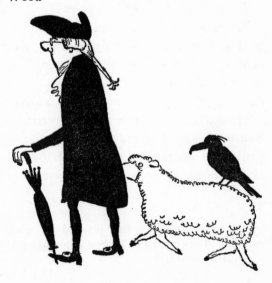

by being the last at something. This was James Hamilton, who was the last in Edinburgh to visit his patients in a sedan chair.[1] In this portable chair, carried by two of his patients who were working out payment of a bill, he made his way for years without ever running out of gas or having a flat.

Still another Scotsman was John Hunter, a comparative anatomist and surgeon. As a boy he was fascinated with the birds and the bees, and not just their sex life. Later he graduated to experiments on hibernating hedgehogs and studied the habits of the cuckoo and the life history of the eel. He dissected everything, from bees to whales, using, we hope, instruments of different sizes. Though he was skillful at dissection, he was a poor lecturer, so nervous before going into the classroom that he often took thirty drops of laudanum. Even then, the students were drowsier than he was. Once so many students cut class that there was only one on hand to hear his lecture. Since he always opened his lecture with "Gentlemen," Hunter, a very honest man, brought in a skeleton and sat it alongside the other student.[2]

Many still believed, with Galen, that the pus which forms in wounds is a good thing. But Hunter, who wrote a treatise on gunshot wounds, was less than

[1] The patients weren't in a sedan chair, he was.
[2] The expression "cutting a class" may have originated in a class in dissection.

enthusiastic. The pro and anti groups, or pus and minus factions, stirred up a good deal of controversy, until Hunter won out with his famous slogan, "Pus must go!" For this he will be remembered, and thanked, by pusterity.[1]

[1] One of my editors, who sickens easily, thinks I have overused the word "pus" above. I have not, however, used it as much as pussible.

Gentlemen!

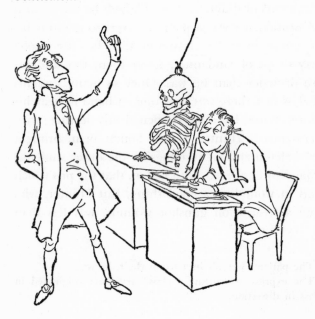

Hunter was always experimenting. Once he injected himself with what he thought was gonorrhea, and it turned out to be syphilis. Another time he purposely delayed treatment after inoculating himself with a pestilential disease, waiting to give the germs a good head start. He finally died, not of any germ-induced disease but of a heart attack.

Obstetrics made great strides in the eighteenth century. For one thing, there was the appearance of the male midwife.[1] His appearance was pretty ridiculous, with his sleeves rolled up and in his arms a tub of hot water. Then too, there was the coming into use of forceps. These were invented by Peter Chamberlen, who told only members of the family about them. The Chamberlens for four generations kept forceps a secret from other obstetricians, carrying them around in a little box with a padlock and a burglar alarm. The patient sometimes tried to steal a look herself, but it was hard to see the things from that angle, and with a black cloth over them.[2]

It is an interesting fact that Peter Chamberlen named both of his sons Peter. Either he had a fixation on the name or forgot he had used it already. In the Chamberlen family there were three medical men

---

[1] The term midhusband never caught on.

[2] Even after they learned about them, some obstetricians declined to use such gadgets. "Fingers were made before forceps," they said scornfully.

named Peter and two named Hugh. No wonder their patients, and the postman, were confused.

Speaking of names, the name of one famous obstetrician is not likely to be forgotten. I refer to William Smellie. The moment he said, "I'm Smellie," you knew this was a man to be reckoned with.[1] Smellie studied in Paris and then settled down in London to teach. Since he could not always be sure of having a baby to deliver at exactly the class hour, he demonstrated with a leather-covered manikin. It was so realistic that when he was through demonstrating

[1] He called his country estate Smyllum, which is Latin for Smellie, and sounds better.

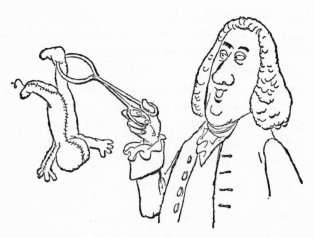

Manikin

and tossed the thing into a corner, students momentarily deplored his manners, bedside or otherwise. By using wooden forceps, Smellie found he could avoid the clicking sound of metal blades, which made him nervous. If an occasional patient complained of splinters, that was a risk that had to be taken.

Finally we come to Edward Jenner and his discovery of a method of vaccinating against smallpox. He found that by giving people cowpox, they wouldn't get smallpox. By the same token, cows that were given smallpox probably wouldn't get cowpox. It is said that if Jenner's method were adopted everywhere, smallpox would disappear from the face of the earth and pock marks would disappear from the faces of people. Vaccination scars, however, would appear on arms, legs, or whatever. Jenner's major work on this subject, *Inquiry into the Causes and Effects of the Variolae Vaccinae,* could have had a catchier title, such as *A Pox on Pox,* but it is widely read in medical circles anyhow. Jenner's name is gratefully remembered, except by small boys with sore arms.[1]

---

[1] These youngsters might think more kindly of Jenner if they knew he was a minor poet and that his poems, such as "Address to a Robin" and "Signs of Rain," are so minor that they don't have to be memorized.

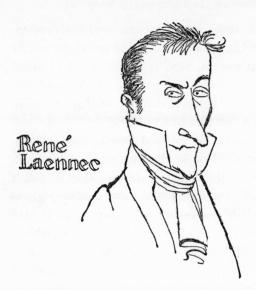

René
Laennec

Chapter Thirteen

INVENTIONS
AND DISCOVERIES

Before discussing medicine of the nineteenth century, let us look briefly at some of the inventions and discoveries that are indispensable to the modern physician, if he remembers to use them.

Though Fahrenheit and Centigrade made their contribution, the originator of the clinical thermometer was an Italian, Santorio Santorio.[1] What he did not explain was how to get a thermometer under the tongue of an uncooperative patient, or how to keep children from crunching it like stick candy. Santorio's first thermometer was administered orally. Had anyone suggested to him the use of the rectum, he would have been embarrassed, as is many a patient

[1] He thoughtfully gave his name twice, to help those who failed to catch it the first time.

today. The rectal thermometer is thought to have come about when a medical student, to whom the professor said "In the mouth," thought he said "In the south."

Physicians had felt the pulse for centuries, but usually had only said "Hmm." The problem in timing the pulse was that watches had no second hand, not even secondhand watches. Santorio invented a pulsilogium, or pulse-clock, but this was thought pretty far out by physicians who were still trying to learn how to shake down the mercury in Santorio's thermometer. It was not until James Currie, a century later, with his Physician's Pulsewatch, that timing the pulse became popular.[1] The Pulsewatch ran for only one minute, and was therefore a great help in reminding the pulse-taker that a minute was up. Occasionally a doctor got his Pulsewatch and his regular watch mixed up and, pulling out his Pulsewatch at a dull party, thought to himself, "Goodness, the time goes slowly tonight!"

Percussion of the thorax as a means of diagnosis was discovered by a Viennese, Leopold Auenbrugger. Auenbrugger, the son of an innkeeper, had often tapped on his father's casks to determine the level of wine.[2] By placing in a row casks of different wine levels, and tapping on first one and then another,

[1] In Queen Victoria's time it was about the only way a young man could hold a young woman's hand without being thought too forward.

[2] Sometimes he merely tapped them, which was one way to be sure the level was lower.

young Auenbrugger could get quite a nice beat, and he was much in demand by the local combos. He is said to have been helped by a "musical ear," which he probably pulled or caused to vibrate in between taps on the casks, and so was virtually a one-man band. But, though he wrote a comic opera, he gave up music for medicine, and while others went around patting people on the back he tapped them on the chest.

Tapping the chest was not enough for some physicians. They wanted to hear everything that was going on inside. For a long time they had been holding their ear against the patient's chest. But though this looked professional, they gained little useful information. Finally a Frenchman, René Laennec, rolled a piece of paper into a cylinder, placed it against the patient's

One-man band

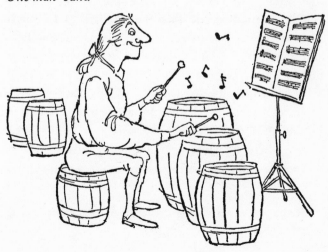

chest, and created the first stethoscope. Since the paper had a tendency to crumple if the doctor leaned on it a little too hard, Laennec next made a stethoscope out of wood. Some later physician thought of metal, which would stay chilled longer, if kept in the refrigerator between calls, and make the patient jump higher when applied.

Nor should we overlook the discovery of oxygen by the French chemist Lavoisier. People had been breathing for years, without knowing why. When Lavoisier pointed out that they were doing this in order to turn oxygen into carbon dioxide, they suddenly felt there was some purpose in life. Ventilation became important, and people threw up windows,[1] let in gusts of cold air, and came down with pneumonia. About the same time Priestley discovered that plants breathe, too, though you can't hear them, and that they turn carbon dioxide into oxygen. Once people learned about this they began to fill their houses with plants, to get rid of the carbon dioxide, and soon were wearing themselves out watering, pruning, and spraying for aphids.

Toward the close of the eighteenth century came the discovery of hypnotism by a Swiss, Franz Anton Mesmer.[2] Mesmer mesmerized people at hypnotic séances, where he wore a lilac-colored suit, played a harmonica, touched his patients with a wand, and

[1] This is not as bad as it sounds.

[2] He put the name Itznang (Switzerland) on the map, but in very small type.

stared into their eyes. The patients meanwhile stood around in tubs full of magnetic compound, holding hands.[1] At the end, as the grand climax, everyone paid through the nose. For a time, in Paris, Mesmer piled up a fortune from his séances, but finally he was forced to get out of town because of practicing without a license, either for medicine or for vaudeville. He was called a fraud or, by those who guessed what was coming, a Freud.

[1] Frankly, they were scared.

Mesmer

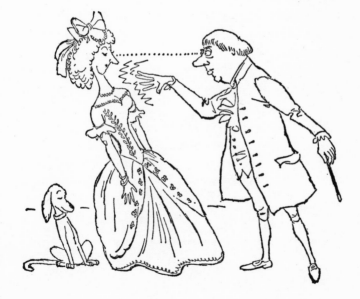

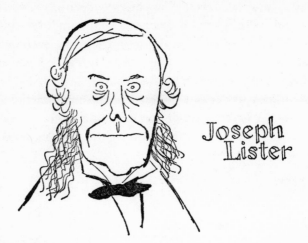

Joseph
Lister

Chapter Fourteen

MEDICINE IN THE
NINETEENTH
CENTURY

Medicine made rapid advances in the nineteenth century. Let us briefly sketch the contributions of some of its outstanding contributors.

Sir Charles Bell discovered that there are two kinds of nerves, sensory and motor. Until Bell's discovery, people were likely to say to one another, "You have a lot of nerve," without distinguishing which kind of nerve it was. Now they could be more specific. Motor nerves developed rapidly with the coming, toward the end of the century, of the motor car.[1] Bell was not

---

[1] It is less frightening to have a car coming toward the end of the century than toward the end of a pedestrian.

only a neurologist but a painter. While other physicians painted wounds, he painted landscapes.

Though there were many capable anatomists, the one who is best remembered is Henry Gray, probably because of his book, *Gray's Anatomy.* This was a very popular book, even though many who picked it up were disappointed that it was not, like Walt Whitman's *Song of Myself,* a detailed description of the parts of the author's body.[1]

Hermann von Helmholtz, the German physiologist, invented the ophthalmoscope, a device that throws a light into the patient's eye, blinding him temporarily. Helmholtz said he had "the great joy of being the first to see a living human retina." One can imagine the scene as Helmholtz jumped up and down with glee, tossing his ophthalmoscope into the air. Having seen far into the eye, he then turned to the ear, becoming a specialist on hearing. But nothing he ever saw, up to and including the eardrum, gave him such a thrill. He tried his best to shine the light from his ophthalmoscope into one ear and out the other, but what with wax and the like he never quite made it.[2]

Then there are several men who will always be remembered because they had a disease named after

[1] Gray and Whitman do, however, have a few things in common. For instance, Gray was a doctor and Whitman was a nurse. And Whitman is known as the good Gray poet.

[2] Or perhaps he did, but could never get over to the other ear in time to see.

them. One was Richard Bright, who gave us Bright's disease.[3] Pointing out that dropsy is the result of kidney trouble, he is responsible for the expression "White clouds in the urine," which is almost as

[3] Well, he didn't exactly give it to us, he gave us the name of it.

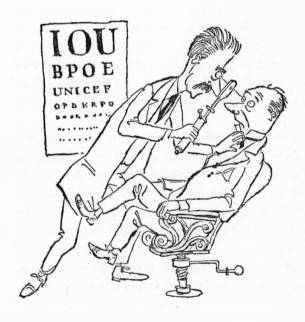

Ophthalmoscope

romantic as "Red sails in the sunset." A colleague of his, Thomas Addison, lent his name to Addison's disease, which might otherwise have been called the suprarenal syndrome. And James Parkinson, with his Parkinson's disease, saved us from having to remember paralysis agitans. It was Parkinson, by the way, who "reported the first case of appendicitis in English." Up to that time cases had been reported, for some reason, in Latin or German, with valuable time lost in translation.

Until Louis Pasteur, it was news when a dog bit a man, because if the dog was mad,[1] the man died of rabies. If the story failed to make the front page, at least it got into the obituary column. But once Pasteur developed a vaccine for rabies, a man had to bite a dog to get any attention, and few were that eager for publicity.

Pasteur discovered that there are millions and millions of bacteria in the air and all around. At first he hesitated to tell people, for fear they would stop breathing. One thing that was full of bacteria was milk. Pasteur found that by heating milk to about 145° he could kill those little creatures, and that is exactly what he did. How the bacteria hated him! Killing bacteria this way is called pasteurization, though to bacteria it is murder. Most important,

[1] Which is different from being angry.

perhaps, was Pasteur's discovery of how to keep food from spoiling, which made it necessary for millions of people to eat leftovers and gave a great boost to the refrigerator industry.

Further advance in bacteriology was made by Robert Koch, who discovered the tubercle bacillus. It is a good thing Koch hadn't come along any earlier, or he would have spoiled many novels, plays, and operas in which the heroine gets paler and paler and weaker and weaker and toward the end coughs into her handkerchief, being a woman of good breeding.[1] Finally the doctor comes out of her bedroom, and from the way he looks you know he has had his last fee from that patient. "There was nothing anyone could do," he says, not having read Koch's paper on tuberculin.

Surgery was furthered by several developments. One came about when Joseph Lister, who believed with Pasteur that bacteria are all over everything, thought that they should be kept from crawling into the wound opened by the surgeon. What Pasteur had done to milk, Lister proposed doing to hands before an operation. When Lister appeared before a gathering of surgeons and suggested, "Maybe you should be sterilized," they thought he was going a little too far. Even when they understood that he merely

[1] Actually it's those dreadful tubercle bacilli that are breeding.

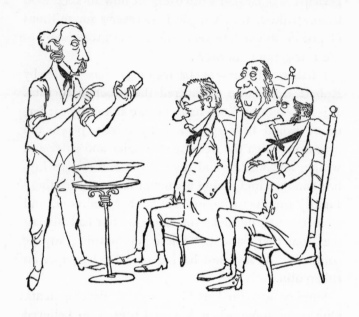

Revolutionary practice

wanted them to boil their hands, they were unco-operative. Finally Lister said that if they just washed their hands, this would help. This revolutionary practice, taken up with some reluctance in England and France, eventually spread to the United States, where it was hailed by the manufacturers of soap. Lister also developed a carbolic acid spray, used as an antiseptic on the wound itself. After surgery, just before closing the wound, Lister would get out his hand pump and, turning to his colleagues, solemnly say, "Let us spray." [1]

As important as antiseptics to the surgeon, and even more important to the patient, was the development of new forms of anesthesia. We have discussed the club of the caveman and the staring eye of Mesmer. Now we come to laughing gas, ether, and chloroform.

Ether was first used by an American, Crawford Long, who applied it to a boy while extracting a tumor from the lad's neck. "That didn't hurt, did it?" he asked when he finished, not because he thought it didn't hurt but because he had been asking the same question for years and couldn't break himself of the habit.

The boy didn't answer, since he was still out cold. Long began to get worried, and thought of putting the tumor back in and pretending nothing had happened. But finally the boy came to, and Long was relieved.[2]

The interesting thing about the first application of laughing gas (nitrous oxide) is that it was employed by Gardner Colton, an American chemist, while one

---

[1] Surgeons did not then wear face masks, but their beards performed much the same function.

[2] Had the boy not come to, Long would still have been relieved, but of his job on the hospital staff.

dentist extracted a molar from another dentist. The dentist with the bad molar had heard enough screams from his patients to be scared to death of having his own tooth extracted. He went around for months with the aching molar before he would let a competitor yank it out. But with laughing gas it turned out to be no trouble at all, except to the dentist who was doing the extracting.

"I wish you would stop laughing a minute," he said, trying to get a good grip on the tooth while the dentist in the chair shook with guffaws.

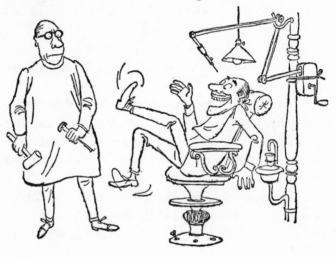

Laughing gas

With the discovery of chloroform, which was poured on a rag and held over the patient's nose, there was a choice of anesthetics. It was ether or.

A final contribution to surgery was made by Wilhelm Konrad Roentgen, who discovered X-rays.[1] With X-rays, surgeons could look inside and see what they were operating for. It was better than just wandering around, hoping.

[1] He called the rays "X" because he couldn't think of just the right word for them. Later someone thought of it: "Roentgen."

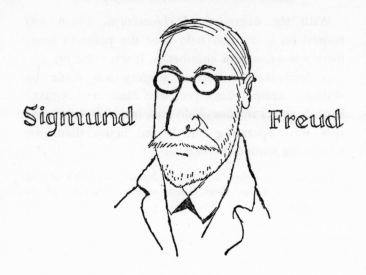

Sigmund Freud

Chapter Fifteen

FREUD

AND PSYCHIATRY

With the advent of psychiatry, medicine got back to the fundamentals with which it began, such as demons which were in the mind and couldn't be cut out with a knife or cured with a pill. Psychiatry affected not only medicine but the national economy, the makers of couches and notebooks having to work overtime to supply the sudden need.[1]

Let us look briefly at the life and works of Sigmund Freud, the father of psychiatry. When Freud came into the world he was covered all over with a heavy

---

[1] Note also the effect of psychiatry on cartoonists, whose favorite theme, next to people marooned on a desert island, became the bearded psychiatrist and his patient.

growth of black hair, which was taken by the super-
stitious folk of the region as a sign of greatness, or at
least of being peculiar. It was subsequently removed
except from his upper lip and chin.

Freud had a beautiful young mother who babied
him, especially while he was a baby. Before he was six
months old he realized that he was in love with her
and hoped he could go on nursing indefinitely. His
father, Jacob Freud, was forty-one when Sigmund was
born and twice as old as his mother (Sigmund's
mother, that is). As a result of a previous marriage,
Jacob had a grandson who was the same age as Sigmund, and it is no wonder young Freud was confused.
He stood outside his parents' locked bedroom door,
thinking evil thoughts and hating his father. By the
time he was in his teens he knew that what he had was
an Oedipus Complex and that life was going to be
complicated.

Freud's childhood marked him for life, leaving a
scar on his psyche. This frustrated him, because when
others opened their shirts or pulled up their trousers
to show their scars, he just stood there helplessly.

Freud became interested in psychoanalysis when
he heard of a patient who was cured of hysteria by
being hypnotized and then asked to recollect how it
all started and tell the doctor the gruesome details.[1]

---

[1] Up to this time the cure for hysteria had been a slap in
the face. This not only stopped hysterics but often started a
fight.

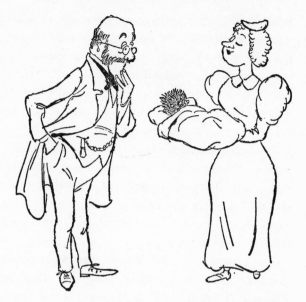

Sign of greatness

Freud replaced hypnosis with free association as a means of resuscitating buried memories, and patients flocked to him, thinking free association meant there was no fee.[1]

Actually it meant that if the patient were given some such word as "rain," this would call to mind the word "umbrella," which in turn would suggest the time the patient left his umbrella in a restaurant and

[1] Were they fooled!

went back to get it and it was gone but noticed a girl who reminded him of his umbrella (perhaps because her ribs were showing) and he struck up an acquaintance and after a short while they were married and he hasn't had a happy day since. So now the patient understands why he becomes hysterical whenever it rains. He thanks the doctor, encouraged by the fact that when it rains the streets are slippery and his wife, who still looks like an umbrella (but now an opened one), may skid into a truck or something. He goes out of the office whistling a merry tune, and henceforth has hysterics only during a prolonged dry spell.

From earliest youth, Freud was plagued by bad dreams. Some of these were so bad that he was ashamed to tell anyone about them. It was therefore a great relief to discover that other people's dreams were every bit as bad as his. When patients were reluctant to tell their dreams to him, he put it on a professional basis and charged them for listening, which reassured them. Actually he would have heard about their dreams for nothing, if necessary, in the interest of medical science and because some of them were really juicy.

One of the first things Freud did was to move a couch into his office, thinking that patients who had not had a dream recently could take a nap and have one right there. Anyhow, they could catch up on their sleep.

Since Freud was the first psychoanalyst, he had no doctor to analyze his own dreams. This forced him to become his own patient, which was difficult but cheaper. He would lie on his couch awhile and then leap up and jot something down, alternating this procedure until he had written such volumes as *The Interpretation of Dreams, Psychotherapy of Everyday Life,* and, as a by-product, *The Autobiography of Sigmund Freud.* Any night he did not have a dream, he felt cheated. Thus he took to raiding the icebox for pickles and cold cuts just to make sure.

By analyzing himself Freud thought he could learn about others, because he considered himself normally abnormal.

According to Freud, the psyche is made up of three parts, the id, the superego, and the ego. The id is the naughty part, lurking in the shadows of the subconscious and thinking up devilish things to do. The superego, which acts like a spoilsport big brother, is always repressing the id and kicking it around, though occasionally the id sneaks by it and causes trouble.[1] As for the ego, it tries to get the superego and the id to be friends, but becomes terribly discouraged.

For Freud, sex was the root of everything. He believed that "sexual impulses date from the cradle," which is something to think about the next time you

---

[1] Or fun, depending on how you look at it.

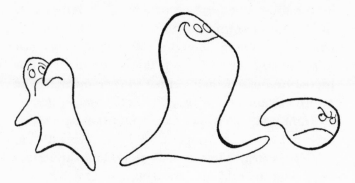

Ego, superego, and id

see a tiny baby slobbering over a teething ring. He also believed that people begin having neuroses soon after they learn to walk. Whether one could avoid a neurosis by never learning to walk he doesn't make clear.

In several of his books Freud writes about the libido, or "sexual hunger." This is what gives people that starved feeling, even between meals. The libido, says Freud, "reaches out from the ego to external objects," and it is a good idea to keep it on a leash, especially around strangers.

Reference was made earlier to the Oedipus Complex, which Freud himself had when he was a boy. The Oedipus Complex was named for a Greek who was about as complex as they come and should have gone to a psychiatrist. Freud, for instance, could have fixed him up after a few visits. Imagine Oedipus on Dr. Freud's couch.

"I'm not normal," Oedipus says, coming right out with it.

"It's normal to think you're not normal," Freud consoles him.

"I killed my father and married my mother. That's bad, isn't it?"

"Almost everybody your age wants to do the same. Only—"

"Only what?"

"Only how would you like it if you had a son and he killed you as soon as he got big enough, and married your widow?"

"That means, in my case, my son would be marrying his grandmother, wouldn't he?"

"Exactly."

"How disgusting. Well, doctor, I may be normal but I'm sick. What have I got?"

"I'm afraid it's an Oedipus Complex, my boy."

"Is there anything I can do for it?"

"Change your name to Ed, or Id. Anyone who has to go around with a name like Oedipus is bound to be on the defensive and try to compensate. You simply overcompensated." [1]

---

[1] In case you don't know, Oedipus is Greek for "swell-foot," by which is meant not a swell foot but a swollen foot. Anyhow, this explains why Oedipus wore sandals instead of shoes.

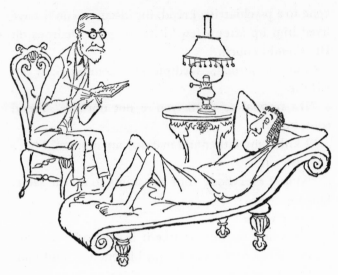

Oedipus on the couch

"Good. What else, doc?"

"Meet some girls your own age. Your mother is old enough to be your mother."

"All right, if you say so. But I'm sorry about what I did to my father."

"Forget it. Everybody makes a mistake now and then."

"I'm better already, doc. You know, I must have been feeling guilty or something."

Oedipus feels fine until he gets Dr. Freud's bill. Fifty dollars for one visit, he thinks, is outrageous.

"But," he muses, "what can you expect from a man who has to go through life with a name like Sigmund? He has to compensate somehow."

Freud lived to be eighty-two, lecturing, writing, interpreting dreams, and asking people searching questions, such as "How's your id?" His work, which has revolutionized medicine, lives on. Less than a hundred years ago Freud was the only psychoanalyst in the world. Now almost everyone is a psychoanalyst, and if you have any bad dreams you had better not talk about them, even in your sleep.

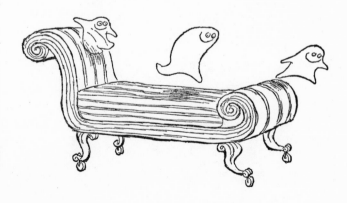

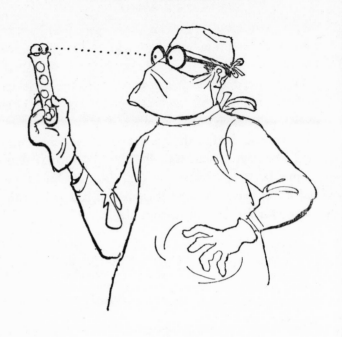

Chapter Sixteen

MEDICINE
TODAY

Probably the ideal of the modern doctor is Sir William Osler, a Canadian who studied in Germany and taught in the United States and England. By moving about briskly, he kept himself in fine trim, all but his mustache.[1] According to his biographer, when he studied in Germany "he sat under Virchow," which must have been humiliating and uncomfortable. When he himself became a teacher, he let his students sit wherever they wished.

Osler, a great practical joker, proved that you needn't be serious to be a successful physician. Once he called up a man named Smith and asked if he would come to lunch to meet Jones. He explained to

[1] Osler had a walrus mustache, among walruses known as an Osler mustache.

Smith that Jones was quite deaf. Then he called up Jones and asked him to come to lunch to meet Smith, explaining that Smith was quite deaf. At lunch, Smith and Jones, both of whom had excellent hearing, leaned forward and yelled at each other, and Osler roared with laughter. When they discovered the joke that had been played on them, it's a wonder they didn't box Osler's ears. Then he might have needed the services of an ear specialist himself.

After teaching for many years at Johns Hopkins, Osler left to teach at Oxford. As his biographer puts it, "He was suffering from overwork, and therefore accepted a call to Oxford as professor of medicine." This says volumes about the difference in teaching loads at Johns Hopkins and Oxford, though the fact that Osler's biographer was a professor at the Johns Hopkins medical school should be taken into consideration.

Osler's picture hangs in the office of many a physician, as a reminder of how lucky one is not to have to wear a high stiff collar like that. And Osler's textbook, *The Principles and Practice of Medicine,* is the Bible of young doctors who are too busy to go to church.

Of recent years there have been remarkable developments in medicine. For instance, when Sir Alexander Fleming discovered penicillin he proved that you should never throw something out just because it is moldy. It may be more valuable than you think. And Salk and Sabin have practically eliminated poliomyelitis, at least in those who remember to drop in for the vaccine. Those who have taken it become so enthusiastic that they come back year after year, and are known as boosters.

While the entertainment world has its Ritz Brothers, Marx Brothers, and Smothers Brothers, the medical world has its Mayo Brothers. If a doctor hasn't a brother to go into practice with, he may have a son, though by the time the son has gone through college, medical school, internship, residency, and training in a specialty, the father is too old to practice any longer. Sometimes a man and his wife are both M.D.'s, with appropriate specialties, the man perhaps being an obstetrician and the wife, taking over from there, a pediatrician. The doctor whose wife is a pathologist may have his dinner cooked over a Bunsen burner, and may have to drink his coffee out of a test tube. More

Over a bunsen burner

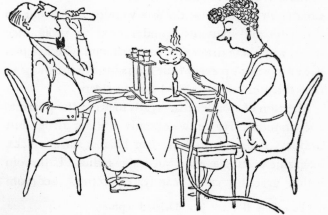

often, though, a doctor marries his nurse or reception-ist, this being the only way he can keep her from leav-ing for another job at a better salary.

With regard to specialization, this has developed considerably of recent years. For a time, for instance, there was the eye, ear, nose, and throat man. Then he became an ear, nose, and throat man, Then a nose and throat man. Now he is a left nostril or a right nostril man. And the end is not in sight.[1] Similarly there is the dermatologist who specializes in moles and won't touch a wart, and can you blame him? And the pediatrician who refuses to treat children who are spoiled, and thinks the ones who are fresh are bad enough. Some believe that specialization is over-done and the family doctor is coming back. But if we had only family doctors, who would treat the bachelor and the spinster? This is something to think about.

Wonder drugs are now in wide use. They are called wonder drugs because doctors wonder which one to prescribe and patients wonder how to pronounce them, why these drugs cost so much, and whether it is better to wake up every four hours during the night to take them or to get a good night's sleep.

Mention of wonder drugs calls to mind the pharma-cist of today. He sells not only wonder drugs but ordinary drugs, as well as razor blades, alarm clocks, magazines, sunglasses, transistor radios, bathroom scales, greeting cards, candy, cigarettes,[2] bedroom

---

[1] Especially if there is a deviated septum.
[2] And remedies to break the cigarette habit.

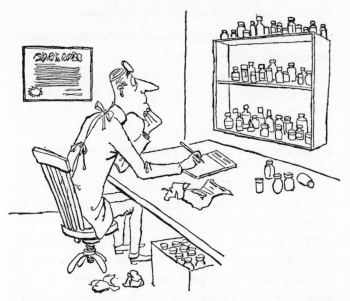

Wonder drugs

slippers, golf balls, and anything else you can think of. The pharmacist himself stays in the prescription room, performing mysterious rites such as scraping the label off a bottle and typing (with one finger, so as to be accurate) a label of his own.

The pharmacist is carefully trained to handle the complicated pharmaceuticals of today. In addition to learning how to pour from a wide-necked bottle into a narrow-necked bottle without spilling (the stuff is expensive), he must have the mathematical training to count as many as 100 pills and an even larger number of trading stamps. Another thing he is taught is to stay safely behind his bulletproof glass partition and let a clerk hand the filled prescription to the customer and tell how much it costs.[1]

But to return to the doctor. Plastic surgery has made great advances, and not only in cutting up plastic.[2] The most important use for plastic surgery is face lifting, some faces having dropped alarmingly.[3] When a woman goes to a plastic surgeon to have her face lifted, a conversation something like this ensues:

"Doctor, do you think my face should be lifted?"

"Something should be done about it, and quickly."

"Will it hurt?"

"Yes, but think of the pain you have given others."

"Will it leave any scars?"

"Only a few small ones, and they will be taken for laugh lines. But I must caution you about one thing."

"What is that, doctor?"

"Don't laugh too hard, or the whole thing will come down again."

There was the famous case of the woman whose face was lifted and she looked young and beautiful again. The only trouble was that she had difficulty with the circulation in her feet. It seems that in firming up her jaw line, the skin had been pulled up from her toes, where it was now too tight. This does not happen too often, however.

[1] It takes a long time to train a registered pharmacist. Clerks are expendable.

[2] Nor is a plastic surgeon a synthetic substitute for the real thing.

[3] I quote from a recent magazine story: " 'You don't mean it!' Ellen said. Her jaw dropped."

Considerable attention has been given by medical researchers to problems of personal hygiene. Thanks to a number of dedicated chemists, often shown at work in their laboratories on TV, powerful anti-perspirants have been developed. These will stop perspiration for as long as twenty-four hours, the sweat glands lying stunned and helpless.[1] Sometimes a woman will telephone her doctor and, without telling the nurse what her trouble is, demand an immediate appointment. All she will say over the phone is, "It's an emergency." When she gets to the doctor she looks at him across the desk, her face ashen.

"Now what is your difficulty?" the doctor asks, expecting his patient to say she has felt a nodule under her left breast and is sure it is cancer.

"I perspire," she blurts out, and then starts sobbing uncontrollably.

The doctor had no idea it was anything so serious. He sees long, difficult treatment ahead, and wishes it were something simple and painless, like a hysterectomy.

Bad breath is another disease which occupies the attention of modern medical science. Thus far the most efficacious remedy seems to be to stop breathing. An important breakthrough was made when it was discovered that by holding the breath a little longer each day, after seventy or eighty years it is possible to get by without any breathing whatsoever. Scientists

---

[1] It might be added that the only thing worse than perspiration is sweat.

are still working on something that will bring quicker results, such as a way to inhale without exhaling.

Reference to inhaling brings to mind the recently established connection between smoking and lung cancer.[1] In view of this, many doctors are recommending various alternatives, such as chewing gum, biting the fingernails, and joining a nudist colony, with no pockets in which to carry cigarettes. As they prescribe this or that, doctors fumble nervously with their cigarette lighters, hoping the patient will stop asking questions and leave, because they haven't had a smoke for twenty minutes and can't stand it much longer.

Some patients who stop smoking get fat. Others get fat whether they smoke or not.

[1] Smoking also contributes to smog, another health hazard.

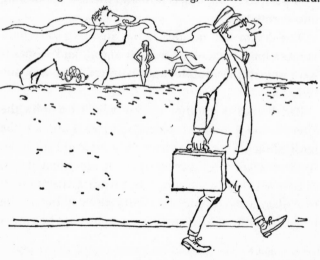

No pockets

"How can I keep down my weight?" is one of the questions most frequently asked of the physician. Actually many people, especially women, keep it down all too well—down around the waist. What they need is to keep it up where it might do some good.

This brings us to diet, which means either eating less or eating only those things you dislike. Diet was no problem in the early days, when people ate a balanced diet not because they knew about proteins and carbohydrates and calories but because a balanced diet was the only kind available. Now, however, physicians are asked to prescribe something, especially if they have forgotten to fix their office scales so they weigh five pounds light. One type of diet is the so-called "crash" diet, which came into being in the lean days after the crash of 1929. This drastic method takes off the pounds rapidly and, if kept up long enough, is a highly successful means of starvation.

Special foods are advocated by some. These include blackstrap molasses, wheat germ, and metal filings, equal parts, a combination which perks up tired blood and puts a sparkle into the eyes.[1] Or there is the pick-me-up of honey, vinegar, and peat moss. The honey sticks to the peat moss, and the vinegar flows freely through the digestive tract, making a man feel as if he is in his salad days. The Orient, and especially China, has recently influenced the eating habits of the Western world. Lotus petals, for instance, have been

[1] The sparkle is caused by the metal filings, which have a way of settling in the cornea.

found to contain all the essential vitamins and minerals. But lotus petals are in short supply, usually being sold out by the time you get to the supermarket. In lieu of anything better from the Mysterious East, there are those who go on a diet of fortune cookies, carefully eating only the small slip of paper inside, made by a Chinese herbalist named No Fat.

There is a difference of opinion about cholesterol, which is said to cause heart attacks. The highest incidence of heart attacks is among doctors at medical meetings, where they get into arguments over whether cholesterol is or is not a bad thing. Doctors who think it is dangerous to have too much cholesterol in the blood are in turn divided into those who believe a non-fat diet will lower the cholesterol and those who

Cause of heart attacks

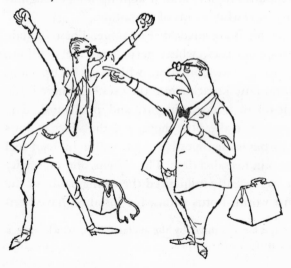

don't. Probably the only way to solve the controversy is by the scientific method of putting one person on a non-fat diet and another on a fatty diet and waiting to see which dies of a heart attack first. The only trouble is that one may die before the other in an auto accident, which would mean starting the experiment all over.[1]

Many remedies are recommended on TV by a man in a white smock with a stethoscope around his neck. He is not an M.D., as you can tell by the careful way he enunciates, and the way he looks you right in the eye while he is reading the script just above the camera. He is also much more certain than an M.D. that the product he recommends will really do the job. The M.D. can, however, learn a great deal from the huckster, for instance how to hold up a bottle and read everything it says on the label without looking at it. He can also learn from the man who plays the part of a doctor in TV serials, for instance how to hire only pretty nurses and how to have patients revive on the operating table after everyone has given them up for dead.

Actually there is enough drama in real life, especially now that artificial organs such as hearts, livers, and kidneys can replace damaged ones. Indeed the time is close at hand when people will carry spare organs, the way they carry spare tires, and have hypo and rubber gloves ready for a quick change by the

[1] The doctor himself may die in an auto accident first, crashing into a car while riding his bicycle to keep fit.

roadside. One of the most dramatic developments is the sewing back on of severed limbs. As yet there has not been an instance of a surgeon's becoming a little confused and sewing on an arm instead of a leg or a leg instead of an arm. But it is only a matter of time.

When surgery is not indicated, the modern doctor, baffled though he may be by the patient's illness, has an easy way out. "It's a virus," he tells the patient. Or, if he has used that one before, "It's an allergy." [1] Patients who undergo skin tests and diet tests for allergy either get well before the testing is completed or die of old age.

A curious development of modern medicine is the so-called "double-blind" technique for testing drugs, a fascinating instance of the blind leading the blind. With this, neither the physician nor the patient knows whether a drug or a placebo is being given— until, that is, the patient either recovers or expires. Some think this technique was borrowed from Russian roulette. As the gambling spirit becomes more pervasive, they foresee slot machines installed in the doctor's office. Instead of dropping coins, the doctor and/or the patient will drop pills. After a pill is dropped and the handle is pulled, the little figures of skulls, medicine bottles, and caduceuses will whirl around. If a solid row of caduceuses comes up, lights will flash, bells will ring, and the doctor and the patient will leap into the air and excitedly embrace

[1] Gray's *Anatomy* has given way to a more literary work, Gray's *Allergy*.

each other, shouting "Jackpot!" and "We've found the cure!"

The "double-blind" slot machine will, of course, be a natural outgrowth of electronic medicine, already well advanced, which permits data to be fed into a computer and a stream of advice to flow out to the physician. The time will come when the physician can sit in his own waiting room, reading a magazine, until he is told what to do. Then, stuffing a wad of computer tape into his little black bag, he will be off on his rounds.

Everyone must have noticed that transfusions are much more common than they were in earlier years. Now if a patient has a slight nosebleed, he is likely to get a pint of blood by transfusion. In the long view of history, it may be that today's transfusions are an

Sick computer

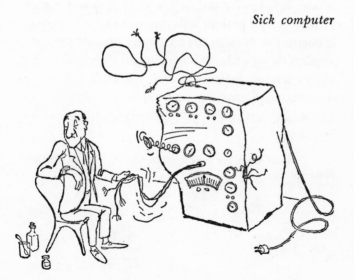

effort by the medical profession to make up for centuries of blood letting.

The increase in medical information has made necessary an ever greater number of medical journals. These are useful around the house to prop open doors and put under leaky flowerpots. Some of the thicker volumes serve nicely to place on a chair and raise small children at the dinner table.[1] Even better than medical journals as a way of being brought up to date on new developments are medical conventions. These are held in central locations like Miami Beach and Honolulu, where doctors go to read papers, there not being time enough to read the paper at home.

With X-rays, wonder drugs, gray ladies, and self-sealing return envelopes for the payment of overdue accounts, medicine has come a long way since the Stone Age. Unlike the doctor awakened at the dawn of history by a patient suffering from a psychosomatic ailment, the modern doctor rouses himself only long enough to prescribe two aspirin and then goes back to his dream of being awarded the Nobel Prize for discovering a cure for the common cold. Or, still better, he leaves the whole thing to his answering service.

[1] In one of them you may even be able to find an article on child raising.

About the Author

RICHARD ARMOUR'S interest in medicine may go back to his boyhood in the family drug store, which he has written about in *Drug Store Days*. His father, grandfather, and grandmother were registered pharmacists, and he himself for a time planned to become a chemist. But thanks to his being born with a screw a little too loose, or a little too tight, he grew up to be one of America's most popular writers of uninhibited humor and satire.

When not writing, he has been involved in scholarly research and teaching. A graduate of Pomona College and a Ph.D. from Harvard, he has taught at seven colleges and universities in various parts of the country and has lectured or been guest-in-residence at numerous others. He has held research fellowships in England, France, and Germany, and has lectured abroad as an American Specialist for the State Department. His irreverent view of higher education will be found in *Going Around in Academic Circles*.

A writer of both verse and prose, Richard Armour has contributed to more than 150 magazines in the United States and England, and this is his thirty-second book. Many of his satires on history and literature, including *It All Started with Columbus, It All Started with Eve, Twisted Tales from Shakespeare, The Classics Reclassified,* and *American Lit Relit,* have been best sellers and have been translated into many languages.

Formerly Dean of the Faculty and Professor of English at Scripps College, he lives in Claremont, California. He is married and the father of a son and a daughter whom, along with the species in general, he dissected in his clinical study of the disease, *Through Darkest Adolescence*.

About the Illustrator

CAMPBELL GRANT, who has illustrated nine of Richard Armour's books, was with Walt Disney for twelve years as a character creator and story man. During World War II he worked with Frank Capra on documentaries. He is the illustrator of many books for children and adults and has done the drawings for the book version of many Disney films. Since 1960 he has been actively interested in archaeology, and has recorded and made paintings of the aboriginal rock paintings in the Santa Barbara mountains and published many articles and a book on the subject. In 1964 he broadened the scope of the study to include the rock art of North America and has completed a definitive book under grants from the National Science Foundation. In his spare time he teaches art at a nearby private school and serves as an art consultant for a publishing house. Living idyllically on a ranch near Santa Barbara, he raises avocados and has a talented writer-wife and four children.